QUACKS and GRAFTERS

By EX-OSTEOPATH

*BEING AN EXPOSÉ OF THE STATE OF
THERAPEUTICS AT THE PRESENT TIME,
WITH SOME REASONS WHY SUCH
GRAFTERS FLOURISH, AND SUG-
GESTIONS TO REMEDY THE
DEPLORABLE MUDDLE*

I

To the
GREAT AMERICAN PUBLIC
is Dedicated
This Book, With Every
Confidence in its Proverbial Common Sense and
Discrimination, and With the Hope of
Having Added a Mite Toward Greater
and Better Things in the
Art of Aesculapius.

PREFACE.

There has been but one other period in the history of medicine when so many systems of the healing art were in vogue. In the seventeenth century, during the Reform Period, following the many epoch-making discoveries, as the blood and lymph circulation; when alchemy was abandoned and chemistry became a science; when Galileo regenerated physics, and zoology and botany were largely extended; when Newton enunciated the laws of gravitation; when cinchona bark, the great febrifuge, was introduced into Europe, and the cell doctrine was founded by Hooke, Malpighi and Grew, the old Hippocratic, Galenic and Arabic systems of medicine were undermined. In that transition period, when the medical profession was trying to adjust its practice with the many new theories, its authoritative voice was lost, and in the struggle for something tangible, innumerable new systems sprang up.

Four systems stood out most prominently—the pietistically colored Paracelsism of Von Helmont, with its sal, sulphur and mercury; the chemical system of Sylvius and Willis, with its acid and alkali theory of cause and cure of disease; the iatro-chemical system, with its fermentation theory; and the iatro-physical system, which contended that health was dependent upon proper adjustment of physical and mechanical arrangements of the body. The old humoral theory of Galen had its adherents, influencing all of the newer systems. And suggestive therapeutics was rampant in most grotesque and fanciful forms. Witchcraft, superstition and cabalism were fostered even at the various European courts. As Roswell Park says in his History of Medicine: "With delightful satire Harvey divided the physicians of the day into six classes—the Ferrea, Asinaria, Jesuitica, Aquaria, Laniaria and Stercoraria—according as their favorite systems of treatment were the administration of iron, asses' milk, cinchona, mineral water, venesection or purgatives."

That history repeats itself is a truism well illustrated in medicine to-day. The new cellular pathology, founded by Virchow and Cohnheim and elaborated by innumerable men since; the discovery of parasitism and the germ theory by Davaine, Pasteur and Koch; antisepsis by Lister; the introduction of anesthesia by Morton, Simpson and Koller; the application of more exact methods in diagnosis by Skoda and others, and many other innovations and discoveries have revolutionized medicine in the nineteenth century. The transition period of to-day is very analogous to that of the seventeenth century.

Suggestive therapeutics has its advocates in the Emmanuel movement, Lourdes water, Christian Science, New Thought, faith cure and psycho-therapy. The uric acid theory is a curious survival of the old chemical system. The iatro-chemical system is the prototype of Metchnikoff's theory of longevity. And, strange to relate, despite the claims of wonderful discovery by A. T. Still and D. D. Palmer, the iatro-physical system of the seventeenth century was more complete as a guide to healing than is Osteopathy and Chiropractics to-day. Verily, there is nothing novel under the solar rays.

That graft in surgery and shystering in internal medicine exists no one in the medical profession denies. It has come so insidiously that the profession itself was taken unawares. However, that sweeping denunciation of the entire profession should follow is unwarranted. Every other profession and calling has its black sheep, and it is the duty of the leaders in each to eliminate them. Elimination, however, cannot come entirely from within. The public has its share of responsibility and duty to perform, and the sooner this is realized, the better for all concerned.

To aid in the work of obtaining better things in therapeutics, the establishment and extension of a national bureau or department of health is imperative. Any effort along this line will hasten the day of rational healing. Preventive medicine will then gradually supplant the present haphazard system of palliation and cure.

And education is the watchword of the day!

G. Strohbach, M.D.

Cincinnati, Ohio, 1908.

PUBLISHERS' NOTE.

Though written in a satirical vein, this book is intended as a warning to the medical profession and the public alike. And, while amusing, the wealth of information and comment on certain abuses in the healing art should lead to serious consideration. This book is published without bias or prejudice toward any school of medicine or system of therapeutics as such. But that quackery and graft are rampant among those who pose as healers has become so apparent that we believe every influence to expose and weed out the pretenders is timely.

The author is an Osteopath who abandoned the practice of Osteopathy after a few years' earnest endeavor, convinced of the untenable position of those professing the practice of this art. He returned to the more congenial profession of teaching. For obvious reasons he publishes this book under a *nom de plume*. He is abundantly fortified with facts to substantiate his criticism.

That his effort may be of some service in clarifying the situation and lead to better therapeutics in the near future, is the sincere hope of

The Publishers.

PART ONE
IN GENERAL

CHAPTER I.

BY WAY OF INTRODUCTION.

The Augean Stables of Therapeutics—The Remedy—Reason for Absence of Dignified Literary Style—Diploma Mills—"All but Holy"—Dr. Geo. H. Simmons' Opinion—American Medical Association Not Tyrannical—Therapeutics of To-day a Deplorable Muddle.

In writing this booklet I do not pose as a Hercules come to cleanse the Augean stables of therapeutics. No power but that of a public conscience awakened to the prevalence of quackery and grafting in connection with doctoring can clear away the accumulated filth.

Like Marc Antony, I claim neither wit, wisdom nor eloquence; but as a plain, blunt man I shall "speak right on of the things I do know" about quacks and grafters. In writing of Osteopathy I claim the right to speak as "one having authority," for I have been on the "inside." As to grafting in connection with the practice of medicine I take the viewpoint of a layman, who for years has carefully read the medical literature of the popular press, and of late years a number of representative professional journals, in an effort to get an intelligent conception of the theory and practice of therapeutics.

I have not tried to write in a professional style. I have been reading professional literature steadily for some time, and need a rest from the dignified ponderosity of some of the stuff I had to flounder through.

I have just read an exposition of the beautiful and rational simplicity of Osteopathy. This exposition is found in a so-called great American encyclopedia that has been put into our schools as an authoritative source of knowledge for the making of intelligent citizens of our children. It is written by a man whose name, like that of the scholar James Whitcomb Riley describes, is "set plumb at the dash-board of the whole indurin' alphabet," so many are his scholarly degrees.

How impressive it is to look through an Osteopathic journal, and see exhaustive (and exhausting) dissertations under mighty names followed by such proof of profound wisdom as, A.M., M.S., D.O., or A.B., A.M., M.D., D.O. Who could believe that a man with all the wisdom testified to by such an array of degrees (no doubt there were more, but the modesty that goes with great learning forbade their display) could be imposed upon by a fad or fake? Or would espouse and proclaim anything that was not born of truth, and filled with blessing and benefaction for mankind?

Scholarly degrees should be accepted as proof of wisdom, but after reading such expositions as that in the cyclopedia, or some of those in the journals, one sometimes wonders if all the above degrees might not be condensed into the one—D.F.

As for dignified style in discussing the subject before me, I believe my readers will agree that dignity fits such subjects about as appropriately as a ten-dollar silk hat fits a ten-cent corn doctor, or a hod-carrier converted into a first-class Osteopath.

While speaking of dignity, I want to commend an utterance of the editor of the *Journal of the American Medical Association*, made in a recent issue of that journal. It was in reply to a correspondent who had "jumped onto" the editor of a popular magazine because in exposing graft and quackery he had necessarily implicated a certain brand of medical practitioners. The man who criticised the editor of the popular magazine impresses a layman as one of that class of physicians that has done so much to destroy the respect and confidence of intelligent students of social conditions for medical men as a class, and in the efficacy of their therapeutic agencies. Although the committee appointed by the great society, of which he is presumably a member, reported that more than half of the medical colleges in this country are utterly unfit by equipment to turn out properly qualified physicians; that a large per cent of these unworthy schools are little better than diploma mills conducted for revenue only, and in spite of the incompetency and shystering that reputable physicians, in self-defense and in duty to the public must expose, this man proclaims that the medical profession is "all but holy" in its care for the souls and minds as well as the bodies of the people. With all respect for the devoted gentlemen among physicians we ask, Is it any wonder that the intelligent laity smile at such gush? And this man goes on to say that "99 per cent. of the practicing physicians of the country belong to this genuine class."

Members of the American Medical Association may think that such discussions are for the profession, and should be kept "in the family." Perhaps they should, and no doubt it would be much better for the profession if many of the things said by leading medical men never reached the thinking public. But the fact remains that the contradictory and inconsistent things said do reach the public, and usually in garbled and distorted form. The better and safer way is, if possible, to see to it that there is no cause to say such things, or if criticisms must be made let physicians be fair and frank with the people, and treat the public as a party deeply concerned in all therapeutic discussions and investigations. And here applies the utterance of the editor of the *Journal of the American Medical Association* that I wanted to commend:

"The time has passed when we can wrap ourselves in a cloak of professional dignity and assume an attitude of infallibility toward the public. The more intelligent of the laity have opinions on medical subjects, often *bizarre*, it must be admitted, but frequently well grounded, and a fair discussion of such opinions can result only in a greater measure of confidence in and respect for the medical profession."

Such honest, fair-minded declarations, together with expressions of similar import from scores of brainy physicians and surgeons in active practice, are the anchors that hold the medical ship from being dashed to wreckage upon the rocks of public opinion by the currents, cross-currents and counter-currents of the turbid stream of therapeutics.

The people have strongly suspected graft in surgery, many of them know it, and nearly all have been taught by journals of the new schools that such grafting is a characteristic of medical schools, and is asserted to be condoned and encouraged by the profession as a whole. How refreshing, then, to hear a representative surgeon of the American Medical Association say:

"The moral standards set for professional men are going to be higher in the future, and with the limelight of public opinion turned on the medical and surgical grafter, the evil will cease to exist."

Contrast such frankness with the gush of the writer who, in the same organ, said 99 per cent. of the medical men were "all but holy" soul guardians, and judge which is most likely to inspire confidence in the intelligent laity.

Right here I want to say that since I have been studying through a cartload of miscellaneous medical journals, I have changed my opinion of the American Medical Association. It is a matter of little consequence to medical men, of course, what my individual opinion may be. It may, however, be of some consequence and interest to them to know that the opinion of multitudes are being formed by the same distorting agencies that formed the opinion I held until I studied copies of the *Journal of the American Medical Association* in comparison with the "riff-raff, rag-tag and bob-tail" of the representative organs of the myriad cults, isms, fads and fancies that "swarm like half-formed insects on the banks of the Nile."

As portrayed by the numerous new school journals I receive, the American Medical Association is a tyrannical monster, conceived in greed and bigotry, born of selfishness and arrogance, cradled in iniquity and general cussedness, improved by man-slaughter, forced upon the people at the point of the bayonet and maintained by ignorance and superstition. Most magazines representing various "drugless" therapies, I found, spoke of the American Medical Association in about the same way. And not only these, but a number of so-called regular medical journals, as well as independent journals and booklets circulated to boost some individual, all added their modicum of vituperation.

When you consider that thousands of Osteopaths (yes, there are several thousand of them in the field treating the people) are buying some one of the various Osteopathic journals by the hundreds every month and distributing them gratis to the people until the whole country is literally saturated, and that other cults are almost as busy disseminating their literature, do you wonder that the people are getting biased notions of the medical profession in general and the American Medical Association in particular? While my faith in the integrity and efficacy of the "new school" remained intact and at a fanatical pitch, my sympathy was with the "independent" journals. The doctrine of "therapeutic liberty" seemed a fair one, and one that was only American. After studying both sides, and comparing the journals, I have commenced to wonder if the man who preaches universal liberty so strenuously is not, in most cases, only working for *individual license.*

I wrote a paper some time ago, out of which this booklet has grown, and sent it to the editor of the *Journal of the American Medical Association.* He was kind enough to say it was full of "severe truth" that should be published to the laity. In that paper I diagnosed the therapeutic situation of to-day as a "deplorable muddle," and I am glad to have my diagnosis confirmed by a prominent writer in the *Journal* of the Association. He says:

"Therapeutics to-day cannot be called a science, it can only be called a confusion. With a dozen dissenting opinions as to the most essential and efficacious therapeutic agents inside the school, and a horde of new school pretenders outside, each with his own little system that he heralds as the best and *only* right way, and all these separated in everything but their attack on the regulars, there certainly is a 'turbidity of therapeutics!'"

And this therapeutic stream is the one that flows for the "healing of nations!" Should not its waters be pure and uncontaminated, so that the invalid who thirsts for health may drink with confidence in their healing virtues?

If the stream shows turbid to the physician, how must it appear to his patient as he stands upon the shore and sees conflicting currents boil and swirl in fierce contention, forming eddies that are continually stranding poor devils on the drifts of discarded remedies, while streams of murky waters (new schools) pour in from every side and add their filth. To the patient it becomes "confusion, worse confounded."

CHAPTER II.

GRAFT AND FAILUREPHOBIA.

The Commercial Spirit—Commercialism in Medicine—Stock Company Medical Colleges—Graft in Medicines, Drugs and Nostrums—Encyclopedia Graft—"Get-Rich-Quick" Propositions—Paradoxes in Character of Shysters—Money Madness—Professional Failurephobia—The Fortunate Few and the Unfortunate Many—A Cause of Quackery—The Grafter's Herald—The World's Standard—Solitary Confinement—The Prisoner's Dream—Working up a Cough—Situation Appalling Among St. Louis Physicians—A Moral Pointed.

This chapter is not written because I possess a hammer that must be used. My liver is sound, and I have a pretty good job. Neither palpation nor "osculation" (as one of our bright Osteopathic students once said in giving means used in physical diagnosis) reveals any "lesion" in my domestic affairs.

However, it doesn't take the jaundiced eye of a pessimist to see the graft that abounds to-day. The grafter is abroad in the land like a wolf seeking whom he may devour, and the sheep-skin (sometimes a diploma) that once disguised his wolfish character has become so tattered by much use that it now deceives only the most foolish sheep. Once a sheep-skin of patriotism disguised the politician, and people fancied that a public office was a public trust. The revelations of the last few years have taught us that too often a public office is but a public steal.

The commercial spirit dominates the age. Nothing is too sacred for its defiling hands to touch. The church does not escape. Preachers accuse each other of following their Lord for the loaves and fishes. Lawyers accuse each other of taking fees from both

16

sides. Leading physicians unhesitatingly say that commercialism is the bane of the medical profession. They say hundreds are rushing into medicine because they have heard of the large earnings of a few fortunate city physicians, and think they are going into something that will bring them plenty of "easy money." Stock company medical colleges have been organized by men whose main object was to get a share of the money these hosts of would-be doctors had to spend. Even the new systems of therapeutics such as Osteopathy, that have boomed themselves into a kind of popularity, have their schools that, to believe what some of them say of each other, are dominated by the rankest commercialism, being, in fact, nothing but Osteopathic diploma mills.

Not alone has graft pervaded the schools whose business it is supposed to be to make capable physicians. The graft that has been uncovered lately in connection with the preparation and sale of medicines, drugs and nostrums is almost incredible when we think of the danger to health and human life involved. The same brand of ghouls who tamper with and juggle medicines for gain, do not hesitate to adulterate and poison food. With their inferior, filthy and "preserved" milk they slaughter the innocents to make a paltry profit. The story Sinclair wrote of the nauseating horrors of slaughter-houses was enough to drive us all to the ranks of vegetarians forever.

Only recently I chanced to learn that even in the business of publishing there is a little world of graft peculiar to itself. I was told by a responsible book man that the encyclopedia containing a learned (?) exposition of the science of Osteopathy is the product of grafters, who took old material and worked in a little new matter, such as the exposition of Osteopathy, to make their work appear up to date to the casual observer. Then, to make the graft worse, for a consideration, it was alleged, a popular publisher let his name be used, and thus thousands were caught who bought the work relying on the reputation of the publisher, who, it appears, had nothing whatever to do with the encyclopedia.

Physicians, school teachers and preachers, all supposedly poor financiers, know about the swarms of grafters who hound them with "get-rich-quick" propositions into which they want them to put their scant surplus of salary or income as they get it. A physician told me he would have been $2,000 better off if a year or two before he had been a subscriber to a certain medical journal that poses as a sort of "watch dog" of the physician's treasury.

Pessimistic as this review may seem, there is yet room for optimism, and, paradoxical as it may sound, men are not always as bad as their business. I know of a lawyer who in his profession has the reputation of being the worst shyster that ever argued a case. No scheme is too dishonest for his use if it will win his case. Yet this man outside of his profession, in his home, and in his society, is as fine a gentleman as you would wish to meet—a model husband and father, a kind and obliging neighbor, a generous supporter of all that is for the upbuilding and bettering of society. Strong case, do you say? I believe our country is full of such cases. And I believe the medical profession has thousands of just such men, men whose instincts are for nobility of character and whose moral ideals are high, but whose business standards are groveling.

They live a sort of "Dr. Jekyll and Mr. Hyde" life, and why? Are they not to blame? And are they not to be classed as scoundrels? Yes—and no. These men are diseased. Their contact with the world has inoculated them with the world's contagion. What is this disease? The diagnosis has been considered simple. So simple that the world has called it commercialism, or money madness, and treated the disease according to this diagnosis without studying it further. May it not be true that, for many cases at least, the diagnosis is wrong? Do men choose the strenuous, money-grabbing life because they really love it, or love the money? I believe thousands of men in professional life to-day, who are known as dollar-chasers, really long for a more simple life, but the disease they have has robbed them of the power to choose "that better part." And that disease is not money madness, but *failurephobia.*

The fear of failing, or of being called a failure, dominates the professional world as no other power could. It claims thousands of poor fellows who were brought up to the active, worth-while life of the farm or of a trade, and chains them to a miserable, sham, death-in-life sort of existence, that they come to loathe, but dare not leave because of their disease, failurephobia.

Success is the world's standard. Succeed in your business or profession, by honest means if you can, but *succeed!* At least, keep up the appearance of succeeding, and you may keep your place in society. It may be known that your business is poor, and that you go to your office and sit in solitude day in and day out, and that you starve and skimp at home, but so long as you keep up the *show,* you are a "professional man!" What mighty courage it takes to acknowledge what everybody else knows, and *quit!* A writer in a medical journal told of a young physician in Boston who put an ad. in a daily paper asking for a job in which a strong man could use the strength a manly man ought to be proud of, to earn an honest living. If men only had the courage, I wonder how many such ads. would appear in the columns of our papers!

An old schoolmate, who is a lawyer in a Western city, told me that of the more than two hundred lawyers of that city, twenty had practically all the law business, and of that twenty a half dozen got the big cases in which there was most money. It is largely so in every city and town. And what applies to the lawyer applies to the physician, though perhaps not to so great an extent. And while the fortunate few get most of the practice, and make most of the money, what are the unfortunate many doing?

Holding on, starving, skimping, keeping up appearances, and, while young, hoping against hope for better days. But when hope long deferred has made the soul sick, and hope itself dies, what then? Keep up appearances, you are a professional man. You can't be a quitter. It would be humorous, were it not so pathetic, to see the old doctor who has dragged along for years, barely eking out a living, put on the silk hat of his more ambitious days and wear it with dignity along with his shiny threadbare trousers and short coat, making a desperate spurt to keep up with the dashing young fellow just out of school.

Failurephobia! Among professional men what a terrible disease it is! I have known it to drive a young man, who might have been happy and useful as a farmer or mechanic, into a suicide's grave. Such cases are not uncommon. Who are the M.D.s whose pictures and glaring ads. appear in those 15-cent papers published in Augusta, Me., and in many daily and even religious papers? Are they men who took to graft and disgraced their profession because they loved that kind of life, and the stigma it brings? Not in many cases. Most of them perhaps come from the ranks of ambitious fellows who lost out in the strife for legitimate practice, but who would not acknowledge failure, so launched into quackery, and became *notorious* if they could not become noted.

Strange as it may seem, the fact that a professional man is a notorious grafter abroad does not necessarily deprive him of social standing at home. I have in mind a man whose smug face appears in connection with a page of loud and lurid literature in almost every 15-cent *Grafters Herald* from Maine to California; yet this man at home was pointed to with pride as an eminently successful man. He wore his silk hat to church, and the church of which he was a valued member was proud of the distinction he gave it. A Western city has an industry to which it "points with pride," and the pictures of the huge plant appear conspicuously placed in illustrated boom editions of the city's enterprising papers. This octopus reaches out its slimy tentacles to every corner of the United States, feeling for poor wretches smitten by disease, real or fancied. When once it gets hold of them it spews its inky fluids around them until they "cough up" their hard-earned dollars that go to perpetuate this "pride of the West."

The most popular themes of the preacher, lecturer and magazine writer to-day are Honesty, Anti-graft, Tainted Money, True Success, etc. You have heard and read them all, and have been thrilled with the stirring words "An honest man is the noblest work of God." The preacher and the people think they are sincere, and go home congratulating themselves that they are capable of entertaining such sentiment. When we observe their social lives we are led to wonder how much of that noble sentiment is only cant after all.

The World's Standard.

The world will say that goodness is the only thing worth while,
But the man who's been successful is the man who gets the smile.
If the "good" man is a failure, a fellow who is down,
He's a fellow "up against it," and gets nothing but a frown.

The fellow who is frosted is the fellow who is down,
No matter how he came there, how honest he has been,
They find him just the same when being there's a sin.

A man is scarce insulted if you tell him he is bad,
To tell him he is tricky will never make him mad;
If you say that he's a schemer the world will say he's smart,
But say that he's a failure if you want to break his heart.

If you want to be "respected" and "pointed to with pride,"
"Air" yourselves in "autos" when you go to take a ride;
No matter how you get them, with the world that "cuts no ice,"
Your neighbors know you have them and know they're new and nice.

The preacher in the pulpit will tell you, with a sigh,
That rich men go with Dives when they come at last to die;
And men who've been like Lazarus, failures here on earth,
Will find their home in Heaven where the angels know their
worth.

But the preacher goes with Dives when the dinner hour comes;
He prefers a groaning table to grabbing after crumbs.
Yes; he'll take Dives' "tainted money" just to lighten up his load.
Enough to let him travel in the little camel road.

That may sound like the wail of a pessimistic knocker, but every
observing man knows it's mostly truth. The successful man is the
man who gets the world's smile, and he gets the smile with little
regard to the methods employed to achieve his "success."

This deplorable social condition is largely responsible for the
multitudinous forms of graft that exist to-day. To "cut any ice"
in "society" you must be somebody or keep up the appearance of
being somebody. Even if the world knows you are going mainly
on pretensions, it will "wink the other eye" and give you the place
your pretensions claim. Most of the folk who make up "society"
are slow to engage in stone slinging, for they are wise enough to
consider the material of which their own domiciles are
constructed.

To make an application of all this, let us not be too hard on the
quack and the shyster. He is largely a product of our social
system. Society has placed temptations before him to get money,
and he must keep up the appearances of success at any cost of
honesty and independent manhood. The poor professional man
who is a victim of that fearful disease, failurephobia, in his
weakness has become a slave to public opinion. He is made to
"tread the mill" daily in the monotonous round to and from his
office where he is serving a life sentence of solitary confinement,

while his wife sews or makes lace or gives music lessons to support the family.

I say solitary confinement advisedly, for now a professional man is even denied the solid comfort of the old-time village doctor or lawyer who could sit with his cronies and fellow-loafers in the shade of the tavern elm, or around the grocer's stove, and maintain his professional standing (or rather sitting). In the large towns and cities that will not do to-day. If the professional man is not busy, he must *seem* busy. A physician changed his office to get a south front, as he felt he *must* have sunshine, and he dared not do like Dr. Jones, get it loafing on the streets. Not that a doctor would not enjoy spending some of his long, lonely hours talking with his friends in the glorious sunshine, but it would not do. People would say: "Doctor Blank must not get much to do now. I see him loafing on the street like old Doc Jones. I guess Doctor Newcomer has made a 'has been' of him, too."

I know a young lawyer who sat in his office for two long years without a single case. Yet every day he passed through the street with the brisk walk of one in a hurry to get back to pressing business. He was so busy (?) that he had to read the paper as he walked to save time to——wait!

Did you ever sit in the office with one of these prisoners and watch him looking out of his window upon prosperous farmers as they untied fine teams and drove away in comfortable carriages? Did you know how to translate that look in his eye, and the sad abstraction of manner into which he momentarily sank, in spite of his creed, which taught him to always seem prosperous and contented? The translation was not hard. His mind was following that farmer out of town and along the green lanes, bordered by meadows and clover bloom, and on down the road through the cool twilight of the quiet summer evening, to where the ribbon of dark green forest, whose cool cadence had called to him so often, changed to groves of whispering trees that bordered the winding

23

stream that spoke of the swimming holes and fishing pools of his boyhood. And on up the road again, across the fertile prairie lands, until he turns in at the gate of an orchard-embowered home. And do you think the picture is less attractive to this exile because it has not the stately front and the glistening paint of the smart house in town? Not at all. The smart house with glistening paint is the one he must aspire to in town, but his ideal home is that snug farmhouse to which his fancy has followed the prosperous farmer.

That picture is not altogether a product of poetic fancy. We get glimpses of such pictures in confidential talks with lawyers and doctors in almost every town. These poor fellows may fret and sigh for change, "and spend their lives for naught," but the hunger never leaves them. Not long ago a professional man who has spent twenty-five years of his life imprisoned in an office, most of the time just waiting, spoke to me of his longing to "get out." His longing had become almost a madness. He forgot the creed, to always appear prosperous, and spoke in bitterness of his life of sham. He said he was like the general of the old rhyme who "marched up the hill and—marched down again." He went up to his office and—went home again, day in and day out, year in and year out, and for what? But *failurephobia* held him there, and he is there yet.

What schemes such unfortunates sometimes concoct to escape their fate! I was told of a physician who was "working up a cough," to have an excuse to go west "for his health." How often we hear or read of some bright doctor or lawyer who had a "growing" practice and a "bright future" before him, having to change his occupation on account of his health failing!

This is not an overdrawn picture. I believe old and observing professional men will bear me out in it. Statistics of the conditions in the professions are unobtainable, but I feel sure would only corroborate my statement. In a recent medical journal was an article by a St. Louis physician, which said the situation among medical men of that city was "appalling." Of the 1,100 doctors there, dozens of them were living on ten-cent lunches at the saloons, and with shiny clothes and unkempt persons were holding on in despair, waiting for something better, or sinking out of sight of the profession in hopeless defeat.

This is a discouraging outlook, but it is time some such pictures were held up before the multitude of young people of both sexes who are entering medical and other schools, aspiring to professional life. And it is time for society to recognize some of the responsibility for graft that rests on it, for setting standards that cause commercialism to dominate the age.

CHAPTER III.

WHY QUACKS FLOURISH.

American Public Generally Intelligent, but Densely Ignorant in Important Particulars—Cotton Mather and Witchcraft—A.B.'s, A.M.'s, M.D.'s and Ph.D.'s Espousing Christian Science, Chiropractics and Osteopathy—Gullibility of the College Bred—The Ignorant Suspicious of New Things—The Educated Man's Creed—Dearth of Therapeutic Knowledge by the Laity—Is the Medical Profession to Blame?—Physicians' Arguments Controvertible—Host of Incompetents Among the Regular Physicians—Report of Committee on Medical Colleges—The "Big Doctors"—Doc Booze—The "Leading Doctor"—Osler's Drug Nihilism—The X-Ray Graft.

In spite of the apparent prevalence of graft and the seemingly unprecedented dishonesty of those who serve the public, there are not wanting signs of the coming of better things. The eminent physician who spoke of the turbidity of therapeutics thought it was only that agitation that precedes crystallization and clarification that brings purity, and not greater pollution. May the seeming bad condition not be due in part also to the fact that a larger number of our American people are becoming intelligent enough to know the sham from the genuine, and to know when they are being imposed upon?

That our American people are generally intelligent we know; but that a people may be generally intelligent and yet densely ignorant in important particulars has been demonstrated in all ages, and in no age more clearly than in our own. We wonder how the great scholar, Cotton Mather, could have believed in and taught witchcraft. What shall we think, in this enlightened age, of judges pleading for the healing (?) virtues of Christian Science, or of college professors taking treatment from a Chiropractor or magnetic healer; or of the scores of A.B.s, A.M.s, M.D.s, Ph.D.s, who espouse Osteopathy and use the powers of their supposedly superior intellect in its propagation?

We can only come to this conclusion: The college education of to-day does not necessarily make one proof against graft. In fact, it seems that when it comes to belief in "new scientific discoveries," the educated are even more easily imposed upon than the ignorant. The ignorant man is apt to be suspicious of new things, especially things that are supposed to require scientific knowledge to comprehend. On the other hand, the man who prides himself on his learning is sure he can take care of himself, and often thinks it a proof of his superior intelligence to be one of the charter members of every scientific fad that is sprung on the people by some college professor who is striving for a medal for work done in original research.

Whatever the reason may be, the fact remains that frauds and grafts are perpetrated upon educated people to-day. In the preceding chapter I tried to tell in a general way what some of the grafts are, and something of the social conditions that help to produce the grafters. I shall now give some of the reasons why shysters find so many easy victims for their grafts.

When it comes to grafting in connection with therapeutics, the layman's educational armor, which affords him protection against most forms of graft in business, seems utterly useless. True, it affords protection against the more vulgar nostrum grafting that claims its millions of victims among the masses; but when the educated man meets the "new discovery," "new method" grafter he bares his bosom and welcomes him as a friend and fellow-scientist. It is the educated man's creed to-day to accept everything that comes to him in the name of science.

The average educated man knows nothing whatever of the theory and *modus operandi* of therapeutics. He is perhaps possessed of some knowledge of everything on the earth, in the heaven above, and in the waters beneath. He is, however, densely ignorant of one of the most important things of all—therapeutics—the matter of possessing an intelligent conception of what are rational and competent means of caring for his body when it is attacked by disease. A man who writes A.M., D.D., or LL.D. after his name will send for a physician of "any old school," and put his life or the life of a member of his family into his hands with no intelligent idea whatever as to whether the right thing is being done to save that life.

Is this ignorance of therapeutics on the part of the otherwise educated the result of a studied policy of physicians to mystify the public and keep their theories from the laity? I don't know. Such accusations are often made. I read in a medical magazine recently a question the editor put to his patrons. He told them he had returned money sent by a layman for a year's subscription to his journal, and asked if such action met their approval. If the majority of the physicians who read his journal do approve his action, their motives *may* be based on considerations that are for the public good, for aught I know, but as a representative layman I see much more to commend in the attitude of the editor of the *Journal of the A. M. A.* on the question of admitting the public to the confidence of the physician. As I have quoted before, he says: "The time has passed when we can wrap ourselves in a cloak of professional dignity and assume an attitude of infallibility toward the public." Such sentiment freely expressed would, I believe, soon change the attitude of the laity toward physicians from one which is either suspicion or open hostility to one of respect and sympathy.

The argument has been made by physicians that it would not do for the public to read all their discussions and descriptions of diseases, as their imagination would reproduce all the symptoms in themselves. Others have urged that it will not do to let the public read professional literature, for they might draw conclusions from the varied opinions they read that would not be for the good of the profession. Both arguments remind one of the arguments parents make as an excuse for not teaching their children the mysteries of reproduction. They did not want to put thoughts into the minds of their children that might do them harm. At the same time they should know that the thoughts would be, and were being, put into their children's minds from the most harmful and corrupting sources.

So in therapeutics. Are not all symptoms of disease put before the people anyway, and from the worst possible sources? If medical men do not know this, let them read some of the ads. in the *Grafter's Herald.* And are the contradictions and inconsistencies in discussions in medical journals kept from the public? If medical men think so, let them read the Osteopathic and "independent" journals. The public knows too much already, considering the sources from which the knowledge comes. Since people will be informed, why not let them get information that is authentic?

Before I studied the literature of leading medical journals I believed that the biggest and brainiest physicians were in favor of fair and frank dealing with the public. I had learned this much from observation and contact with medical men. After a careful study of the organ of the American Medical Association my respect for that organization is greatly increased by finding expressions in numbers of articles which show that my opinion was correct. In spite of all the vituperation that is heaped upon it, and in spite of the narrowness of individual members, the American Medical Association does seem to exist for the good of humanity. The strongest recommendation I have found for it lies in the character of the schools and individuals who are most bitter against it. It is usually complimentary to a man to have rascals array themselves against him.

There are many able men among physicians who feel keenly their limitations, when they have done their best, and this class would gladly have their patients understand the limitations as well as the powers of the physician. In sorrow and disgust sometimes the conscientious physician realizes that he is handicapped in his work to either prevent or cure disease, because he has to work with people who have wrong notions of his power and of the potency of agencies he employs. With shame he must acknowledge that the people hold such erroneous ideas of medicine, not because of general ignorance, but because they have been intentionally taught them by the army of quacks outside and the host of grafters and incompetents *inside* the regular medical profession.

Incompetent physicians, to succeed financially (and that is the only idea of success incompetents are capable of appreciating), must practice as shysters. They fully understand how necessary it is to the successful working of their grafts to keep the people in ignorance of what a physician may legitimately and conscientiously do.

Our medical brethren who preach the "all but holy" doctrine, and want to maintain the "attitude of infallibility toward the public," will disagree with me about there being "a host" of incompetents in the regular school of medical practice. I shall not ask that they take the possibly biased opinion of an ex-Osteopath, but refer them to the report of the committee appointed by the American Medical Association to examine the medical colleges of the United States as to their ability to make competent physicians. "One-half of all the medical schools of our country are utterly unfit to turn out properly qualified physicians, and many of them are so dominated by commercialism that they are but little better than diploma mills"! That's what the committee said.

It has been argued that the capable physician need not fear the incompetent pretender, for, like dregs, he must "settle to the bottom" and find his place. This might be true if the people had correct notions of the true theory of therapeutics. As it is, the scholarly, competent physician knows (and intelligent laymen often know) that the pretenders too often are the fellows who get the reputations of being the "big doctors." Why? I think mainly because, being ignorant, they practice largely as quacks, and by curing (?) all kinds of dangerous (on their own diagnosis) diseases quickly, "breaking up" this and "aborting" that unbreakable and unabortable disease (by "hot air" treatment mainly), they place the whole system upon such a basis of quackery that the deluded masses often pronounce the best equipped and most conscientious physician a "poor doctor," because he will not pretend to do all that the wind-jamming grafter claims *he has* done and *can* do.

Here is a case in point which I know to be true. The farce began some years ago in a small college in Oregon. A big, awkward, harmless-looking fellow came to the college one fall and entered the preparatory department. At the end of the year, after he had failed in every examination and shown conclusively that he had no capacity to learn anything, he was told that it was a waste of time for him to go to school, and they could not admit him for another year. Was he squelched? Not he. The fires of ambition yet burned in his breast, and the next year he turned up at a medical college. I presume it had the same high educational requirements for admission that some other medical colleges have, and enforced them in about the same way. At any rate he met the requirements ($$$), and pursued his medical researches with bright visions of being a doctor to lure him on. But his inability to learn anything manifested itself again, and, presumably, his money gave out. At any rate he was sent away without a diploma. Still the fire of ambition was not extinguished in his manly bosom. Regulations were not strict in those days, so he went to a small town, wore fine clothes, a silk hat and a pompous air, and—within a short time was being called for forty miles around

31

to "counsel little doctors" in their desperate cases. Such cases are all too common, as honest physicians know.

How humiliating to the conscientiously equipped doctor to hear people say of a man who never had more brains than he needed, and had hopelessly muddled what he had by using his own dope and stimulants: "I tell you Doc Booze is the best doctor in town yet when he's half sober!" Strange, isn't it, that in many communities people have an idea that an inclination on the part of a physician toward whisky or dope indicates some peculiar mental fitness for a doctor? "Poor fellow, he formed the habit of taking stimulants to keep up when he had to go night and day during the big typhoid epidemic, you know." For what per cent. of cases of medical dipsomaniacs this constitutes a stock excuse, only medical men know. As an Osteopathic physician I was never rushed so that I felt the necessity for "keeping up on stimulants." If I had been, to be consistent, I should have had to stimulate (?) mechanically, of course.

Not only do shysters and pretenders abuse the confidence of the masses in matters of diagnosis and medication, but of late years they are working another species of graft that is beginning to react against the profession. This graft consists in the over-use of therapeutic appliances that are all right in their place when legitimately used.

By what standard is the physician judged by the people who enter his office? It used to be the display of medical literature. Sometimes some of it was pseudo-medical literature. Did you ever know a shyster to pad his library with Congressional reports? I have. The literature used to be conspicuously placed in the waiting-room, with a ponderous volume lying open on the desk.

Have you a "leading doctor" in your town? Often he is not only in the lead but has flagged all the others at the quarter post—put them all into the "has been" class. What an elegant office he has!

Plush rugs and luxurious couches in the waiting-room. Double doors into the private and operating-rooms, left open when not in actual use to give impressive glimpses of glass cases filled with glittering instruments, any one of which would give the lie to Solomon's declaration that "there is nothing new under the sun." An X-ray machine fills a conspicuous corner. In the same room are tanks, tubes, inhalers, hot-air appliances, vibrators, etc. One full side of the room is filled with shelves that groan under a load of the medicines he "keeps and dispenses." What are all of these hundreds of bottles for if it is true, as many of our greatest physicians say, that a comparatively few people are benefited by drugs? These numerous bottles may contain placebos. I do not know as to that, but I do know something of the impression such a display makes on the mind of an intelligent layman. The query in his mind is how much of that entire display is for its legitimate effect on the minds of the patients, and how much of it is to impress the people with the powers of this physician, with his "wonderful equipment" to cope with all manner of disease?

If there is any doubt in the minds of physicians that laymen do know and think well over the sayings of drug nihilists, let them talk with intelligent people and hear them quote from the editorial page of a great daily such sentiments as this (from the Chicago *Record-Herald*):

"Prof. William Osler, the distinguished teacher of medicine, who was taken from this country a few years ago to occupy the most important medical chair in Great Britain, has shocked his profession repeatedly by his pronouncements against the use of drugs and medicines of almost every kind. Only a few days ago he made an address in which he declared that even though most physicians will be deprived of their livelihood, the time must soon come when sound hygienic advice for the prevention of disease will take the place of the present system of prescription and *pretense of cure*. The most able physicians agree with him, even when they are not frank enough to express themselves to the same effect."

Medical men need not think, either, that the people who happened to read the editorial pages referred to are the only ones who know of that declaration from Osier. Osteopathic journals, Christian Science journals, health culture journals, and all the riff-raff of journals published as individual boosters, are ever on the watch for just such things, and when they find them they "roll them under their tongue as sweet morsels." They chew them, as Carleton says, with "the cud of fancy," and hand them along as latest news to tens of thousands of people who are quick to believe them.

Going back to the physician who has the well-equipped office, is he a grafter in any sense? I shall not give my opinion. Perhaps every thing he has in the office is legitimate. In the opinion of the masses of that community he is the greatest doctor that ever prescribed a pill or purloined an appendix. Taking the word of the physicians whom he has put into the "has been" class for it, he is the greatest fake that ever fooled the people. Most of those outclassed doctors will talk at any time, in any place, to any one, of the pretensions of this type of physician. They will tell how he dazzles the people with his display of apparatus "kept for show;" how he diagnoses malarial fever as typhoid, and thus gets the reputation of curing a larger per cent. of typhoid than any other doctor in town; how he gets the reputation of being a big surgeon by cutting out healthy ovaries and appendices, and how he assists with his knife women who do not desire Rooseveltian families. They point to the number of appendectomies he has performed, and recall how rare such cases were before his advent, and yet how few people died with appendicitis. Is it to be wondered that intelligent laymen sometimes lose faith in and respect for the profession of medicine and surgery?

To show that people may be imposed upon by illegitimate use of legitimate agencies I call attention to an article published recently in the *Iowa Health Bulletin*. The Iowa Medical Board is winning admiration from many by conducting a campaign to educate the people of the State in matters pertaining to hygienic living. In line with this work they published an article to correct the erroneous idea the laity have of the X-ray. They say:

"The people think that with the X-ray the doctor can look right into the body and examine any part or organ and tell just what is the matter with it, when the fact is all that is ever seen is a lot of dim shadows that even the expert often fails to understand or recognize."

Why do the people have such erroneous conceptions of the X-ray? Is it accidental, or the result of their innate stupidity? Certainly it is not. The people have just such conceptions of the X-ray as they receive from the faker who uses it as he uses his opiates and stimulants—to get an effect and give the people wrong ideas of his power.

A lady of a small town who was far advanced in consumption was taken to a city to be examined by a "big doctor" who possessed an X-ray. He "examined" her thoroughly by the aid of the penetrating light made by his machine, and sent them home delighted with the assurance that his wonderful instrument revealed no tuberculosis. He assured her that if she would avail herself of his superior skill she might yet be restored to health. She died within a year from the ravages of tuberculosis.

A boy of four had an aggravated attack of bronchitis. His symptoms were such that his parents thought some object might have lodged in his trachea. A noted surgeon who had come one hundred miles from a hospital to see another case was consulted. He told the parents that the boy had sucked something down his windpipe, and advised them to bring him to the hospital for an operation. They did so, and a $100 incision was made after the X-ray had located (?) an object lodged at the bifurcation of the trachea. The knife found nothing, however, and the boy still had his bronchitis, and the parents had their hospital and surgeon's bills, and, incidentally, their faith in the X-ray somewhat shattered.

The X-rays, Finsen rays, electric light and sunlight have their place in therapy. Informed people do not doubt their efficacy. However, the history of the use of these agents is a common one. A scientist, after possibly a lifetime of research, develops a new therapeutic agent or a new application of some old agent. He gives his findings to the world. Immediately a lot of half-baked professional men seize upon it, more with the object of self-laudation and advertisement than in a true scientific spirit. Serious study in the application of the new agent is not thought of. The object is rather to have the reputation of being an up-to-snuff man. The results obtained are not what the originator claimed, which is not to be wondered at. The abuse of the remedy leads to abuse of the originator, which is entirely unfair to both.

This state of affairs has grown so bad that scientists now are beginning to restrict the application of their discoveries to their own pupils. A Berlin *savant*, assistant to Koch, has developed the use of tuberculin to such a point as to make it one of the most valuable remedies in tuberculosis. It is manufactured under his personal supervision, and sold only to such physicians as will study in his laboratory and show themselves competent to grasp the principles involved.

CHAPTER IV.

TURBID THERAPEUTICS.

An Astounding Array of Therapeutic Systems—Diet—Water—Optics—Hemotherapy—Consumption Cures—Placebos—Inconsistencies and Contradictions—Osler's Opinion of Appendicitis—Fair Statement of Limitations in Medicine Desirable.

To be convinced that therapeutics are turbid, note the increasing numbers of diametrically opposed schools springing up and claiming to advocate the only true system of healing. Look at the astounding array:

Allopathy, Homeopathy, Eclecticism, Osteopathy, Electrotherapy, Christian Science, Emmanuel movement, Hydrotherapy, Chiropractics, Viteopathy, Magnetic Healing, Suggestive Therapeutics, Naturopathy, Massotherapy, Physio-Therapy, and a host of minor fads that are rainbow-hued bubbles for a day. They come and go as Byron said some therapeutic fads came and went in his day. He spoke of the new things that astounded the people for a day, and then, as it has been with

"Cowpox, tractors, galvanism and gas,
The bubble bursts and all is air at last."

One says he has found that fasting is a panacea. Another says: "He is a fool; you must feed the body if you expect it to be built up."

One says drinking floods of water is a cure-all. Another says the water is all right, but you must use it for the "internal bath." Still another agrees that water is the thing, but it must be used in hot and cold applications.

One faker says *he* has found that most diseases are caused by defective eyes, and proposes to cure anything from consumption to ingrown toe-nails with glasses. Another agrees that the predisposing cause of diseases is eye strain, but the first fellow is irrational in his treatment. Glasses are unnatural and therefore all wrong. To cure the eyes use his wonderful nature-assisting ointment; that goes right to the optic nerve and makes old eyes young, weak eyes strong, relieves nerve strain and thereby makes sick people well.

Another has found that "infused" blood is the real elixir of life. He reports 100 per cent. of twenty cases of tuberculosis cured by his beneficent discovery. I wonder why we have a "Great White Plague" at all; or why we have international conventions to discuss means of staying the ravages of this terrible disease; or why State medical boards are devoting so much space in their bulletins to warn and educate the people against the awful fatality of consumption, when to cure it is so easy if doctors will only use blood?

Even if the hemotherapist does claim a little too much, there is yet no cause for terror. A leading Osteopathic journal proclaims in large letters that the Osteopath can remove the obstruction so that nature will cure consumption.

Christian Scientists and Magnetic Healers have not yet admitted their defeat, and there are many regulars who have not surrendered to the plague. So the poor consumptive may hope on (while his money lasts). Our most conscientious physicians not only admit limitations in curing tuberculosis, but try to teach the people that they must not rely on being "cured" if they are attacked, but must work with the physician to prevent its contagion. The intelligent layman can say "Amen" to that doctrine.

The question may be fairly put: "Why not have more of such frankness from the physician?" The manner in which the admissions of doctors that they are unable to control tuberculosis with medicine or surgery alone has been received by intelligent people should encourage the profession. It would seem more fair to take the stand of Professor Osler when he says that sound hygienic advice for the prevention of diseases must largely take the place of present medication and pretence of cure.

As a member of the American Medical Association recently said, "The placebo will not fool intelligent people always." And when it is generally known that most of a physician's medicines are given as placebos, do you wonder that the claims of "drugless healers" receive such serious consideration?

The absurd, conflicting claims of quack pretenders are bad enough to muddle the situation and add to the turbidity of therapeutics; but all this is not doing the medical profession nearly as much harm, nor driving as many people into the ranks of fad followers, as the inconsistencies and contradictions among the so-called regulars.

This was my opinion before I made any special study of therapeutics, and while studying I found numbers of prominent medical men who agree with me. One of them says that the "criticisms," quarrels, contradictions, and inconsistencies of medical men are doing more to lower the profession in the estimation of the intelligent laity and to cause people to follow the fads of "new schools" than all else combined.

Think for a moment of some of these inconsistencies and contradictions. One doctor in a town tells the people that he "breaks up" typhoid fever. His rival, perhaps from the same

39

college, tells the people that typhoid must "run its course" and cannot be broken up, and that any man who claims the contrary is a liar and a shyster. One surgeon makes a portion of the people believe he has saved dozens of lives in that community by surgical operations; the other physicians of the town tell the people openly, or at least hint, that there has been a great deal of needless butchery performed in that community in the name of surgery. And then the people see editorials in the daily press about the fad of having operations performed, and read in their health culture or Osteopathic journals from articles by the greatest M.D.s, in which it is admitted that surgery is practiced too largely as a graft. Professor Osler is quoted as saying:

"Surgeons are finding altogether too many cases of appendicitis these days. Appendicitis is becoming so common and so easily detected that the physician's wife can diagnose a case of it over the telephone."

One leading physician says medical treatment has little beneficial effect on pneumonia; another claims to be able to cure it, and lets the friends of his patient rely entirely on his medicine in the most desperate cases. Another says the main reliance should be heat. Another says ice-packs. Another says Antiphlogistine. Another says, "All those clay preparations are frauds, and the only safe way to treat pneumonia is by blood letting." Thus it goes, and this is only a sample of contradictions that arise in the treatment of diseases.

Nor is the above an overdrawn picture. Most of it was from the journal of the editor who said he refused to send it to a layman who had sent his money in advance. But all that same stuff has been hashed and rehashed to the people through the sources I have already mentioned. There are not only these evidences of inconsistencies to edify (?) the people, but constantly recurring examples of incompetency and pretensions.

There is no doubt a middle ground in all this, but it is not evident to the casual observer. If the true physician would honestly admit his limitations to the intelligent laity, much of this muddle would be avoided. While by such a course he may occasionally temporarily lose a patient, in the end both the public and profession would gain. The time has gone by to "assume an air of infallibility toward the public."

CHAPTER V.

THE EXPERT WITNESS AND PROPRIETARY MEDICINES.

The "Great Nerve Specialist"—The Professional Witness a Jonah—The "Railway Spine"—Is it Lack of Fairness and Honesty or Lack of Skill and Learning?—Destruction of Fine Herds of Cattle Without Compensation—Koch's Dictum and Denial—Koch's Tuberculin—The Serum Tribe—Stupendous Sale of Nostrums—Druggist's Arguments—Use of Proprietary Medicines Stimulates Sale of Nostrums.

I wonder what the patrons of the sanitarium of the "great nerve specialist" thought of his display of knowledge of the nervous system when he was on the witness stand in a recent notorious case? A lawyer tangled him up completely, and showed that the doctor had no accurate knowledge of the anatomy of the nervous system. When asked the origin of the all-important pneumogastric nerve, he *thought* it originated in a certain segment of the spinal cord! This noted "specialist" was made perfectly contemptible, and the whole profession must have blushed in shame at the spectacle presented. And that spectacle was not unnoticed by the intelligent laity.

The professional witness has in most cases been a Jonah to the profession. It is about as easy to get the kind of testimony you want from a professional witness in a suit for damages for personal injuries as it is to get a doctor's certificate to get out of working your poll-tax, or a certificate of physical soundness to carry fraternal life insurance.

Let me recall the substance of a paper read a few years ago by perhaps the greatest lawyer in Iowa (afterward governor of that State). He told of a trial in which he had examined and cross-examined ten physicians. It was a trial in which suit was brought to recover damages for personal injury, a good illustration of the "railway spine." One physician testified that the patient was afflicted with sclerosis of the spinal cord; another said it was a plain case of congestion of the cord; another diagnosed degeneration of the cord; yet another said it was a true combination of all the conditions named by the first three. They all said there was atrophy of the muscles of the left leg, and predicted that complete paralysis would surely supervene.

On the other side five noted physicians testified as positively that neither the spinal cord nor any nerve was injured; that there was no sign of atrophy or loss of power in the leg; and they seemed to think the disease afflicting the patient was due to a fixed desire to secure a verdict for large damages from the railway company. One eminent specialist made oath that the electrical test showed the partial reaction of degeneration; another as famous challenged him to make the test again in the presence of both. After it was made this second specialist went before the jury and positively declared that there was no trace whatever of the reaction of degeneration, and that the muscles responded to the current precisely as healthy muscles should.

Then this eminent attorney adds: "If the instances of such diversity were rare they might pass unnoticed, but they occur and re-occur as often as physicians are called to the temple of justice for the expression of opinions."

The lay mind imputes this clash of opinions either to lack of fairness and honesty or lack of skill and learning. In either case the profession suffers great injury in the estimation of those who should have for it only the profoundest admiration and the most implicit faith. Again I ask, Is it any wonder people have lost implicit faith when they read many reports of similar cases rehashed in the various yellow journals put into their hands?

Farmers submitted with all possible grace to the decrees of science when, by the authority of such a great man as Koch, their fine herds of cattle were condemned as breeders and disseminators of the great white plague and destroyed without compensation. But how do you think these same farmers feel when they read in yellow journals that Koch has changed his mind about bovine and human tuberculosis being identical, and has serious doubts about the one contracting in any way the disease of the other. People read with renewed hope the glowing accounts of the wonderful achievements of Dr. Koch in finding a destroyer for the germ of consumption. Somehow time has slipped by since that renowned discovery, with consumption still claiming its victims, and many physicians are saying "Koch's great discovery is proving only a great disappointment."

Drugless therapy journals are continually pouring out the vials of their wrath upon vaccination, antitoxin and all the serum tribe, and their vituperation is even excelled by vindictive denunciations of the same things by the individual boomer journals that flood the land.

Another bitter contention that is confusing some, and disgusting others, is the acrimonious strife between users and non-users of proprietary medicines. This usually develops into a sort of "rough house" affair, the druggist mixing up as savagely as the doctors before the fight is finished. I know nothing of the rights or wrongs of the case nor of the merits or demerits of proprietary medicines, but I do know this, however: The stupendous sale of nostrums that in 1907 represented a sum of money sufficient to have provided every practitioner of medicine in the United States with a two thousand dollar salary, has been helped by the use of proprietary medicines. I am aware that my position is likely to be called in question by many physicians. But they should hear druggists arguing with people who hesitate about buying patent medicines because their physicians tell them they should seldom take medicine unless prescribed by a doctor. They would hear

44

him say: "Your doctor gives you medicines that are put up in quantities for him just as these patent medicines are put up for us." He then produces literature and proves it—at least beyond the refutation of the patient. Physicians would then realize, perhaps, how the use of proprietary medicines stimulates the sale of nostrums.

CHAPTER VI.

FAITH CURE AND GRAFT IN SURGERY.

Suggestive Therapeutics Chief Stock in Trade—Advice of a Medical College President—Disease Prevention Rather than Cure—Hygienic Living—The Medical Pretender—"Dangerous Diagnosis" Graft—Great Flourish of Trumpets—No "Starving Time" for Him—"Big Operations"—Mutilating the Human Body—Dr. C. W. Oviatt's Views—Dr. Maurice H. Richardson's Incisive Statements—Crying Need for Reform—Surgery that is Useless, Conscienceless and for Purely Commercial Ends—Spirit of Surgical Graft, Especially in the West—Fee-Splitting and Commissions—A Nation of "Dollar-Chasers"—The Public's Share of Responsibility—Senn's Advice—The "Surgical Conscience."

I think we have enough before us to show why intelligent people become followers of fads. Seeing so many impositions and frauds, they forget all the patient research and beneficent discoveries of noble men who have devoted their lives to the work of giving humanity better health and longer life. They are ready at once to denounce the whole medical system as a fraud, and become victims of the first "new system" or healing fad that is plausibly presented to them.

And here a question arises that is puzzling to many. If these systems are fads and frauds, why do they so rapidly get and retain so large a following among intelligent people? The answer is not hard to find. The quacks of these fad schools get their cures, as every intelligent doctor of the old schools knows, in the same way and upon the same principle that is so important a factor in medical practice, i. e., *faith cure*—the psychic effect of the thing done, whether it be the giving of a dose of medicine, a Christian

Science pow-wow, the laying on of hands, the "removal of a lesion" by an Osteopath, the "adjustment" of the spine by a Chiropractor, or what not.

The principles of mind or faith cure are legitimately used by the honest physician. Suggestive therapeutics is being systematically studied by many who want to use it with honesty and intelligence. They realize fully that abuse of this principle figures largely in the maintenance of the shysters in their own school, and it is the very foundation of all new schools and healing fads. The people must be made to know this, or fads will continue to flourish.

The honest physician would be glad to have the people know more than this. He would be glad to have them know enough about symptoms of diseases to have some idea when they really need the help of a physician. For he knows that if the people knew this much all quacks would be speedily put out of business.

I wonder how many doctors know that observing people are beginning to suspect that many physicians regulate the number of calls they make on a patient by motives other than the condition of the patient—size of pocketbook and the condition of the roads, for instance. I am aware that such imputation is an insult to any physician worthy of the name, but the sad fact is that there are so many, when we count the quacks of all schools, unworthy of the name.

The president of a St. Louis medical college once said to a large graduating class: "Young men, don't go to your work with timidity and doubts of your ability to succeed. Look and act your part as physicians, and when you have doubts concerning your power over disease *remember this*, ninety-five out of every hundred people who send for you would get well just the same if they never took a drop of your medicine." I have never mentioned this to a doctor who did not admit that it is perhaps true. If so, is there not enough in it alone to explain the apparent success of quacks?

Again I say there are many noble and brainy physicians, and these have made practically all the great discoveries, invented all the useful appliances, written all the great books for other schools to study, and they should have credit from the people for all this, and not be misrepresented by little pretenders. Their teachings should be applied as they gave them. The best of them to-day would have the people taught that a physician's greatest work may be done in preventing rather than in curing disease. Physicians of the Osler type would like to have the people understand how little potency drugs have to cure many dangerous diseases when they have a firm hold on the system. They would have some of the responsibility removed from the shoulders of the physician by having the people understand how much they may do by hygienic living and common-sense use of natural remedies.

But the conscientious doctor too often has to compete with the pretender who wants the people to believe that *he* is their hope and their salvation, and in him they must trust. He wants them to believe that he has a specific remedy for every disease that will go "right to the spot" and have the desired effect. People who believe this, and believe that without doctoring the patient could never get well, will sometimes try, or see their neighbors try, a doctor of a "new school." When they see about the same proportion of sick recover, they conclude, of course, that the doctor of the "new school" cured them, and is worthy to be forever after intrusted with every case of disease that may arise in their families.

This is often brought about by the shyster M.D. overreaching himself by diagnosing some simple affection as something very dangerous, in order to have the greater credit in curing it. But he at times overestimates the confidence of the family in his ability. They are ready to believe that the patient's condition is critical, and in terror, wanting the help of everything that promises help, call in a doctor of some "new school" because neighbors told how he performed wonderful cures in their families. When the patient recovers speedily, as he would have done with no treatment of any kind, and just as the shyster M.D. thought he would, the glory and credit of curing a "bad case" of a "dangerous disease" go to the new system instead of redounding to the glory of Dr. Shyster, as he planned it would.

Is it any wonder true physicians sometimes get disgusted with their profession when they see a shyster come into the town where they have worked for years, patiently and conscientiously building up a legitimate practice that begins to promise a decent living, and by such quack methods as diagnosing cases of simple fever, such as might come from acute indigestion or too much play in children, as something dangerous, typhoid or "threatened typhoid," or cases of congestion of the lungs as "lung fever," and by "aborting" or "curing" these terrible diseases in short order and having his patients out in a few days, jumps into fame and (financial) success at a bound? Because the typhoid (real typhoid) patients of the honest doctor lingered for weeks and sometimes died, and because frequently he lost a case of real pneumonia, he made but a poor showing in comparison with the new doctor. "He's just fresh from school, you know, from a post-graduate course in the East." Or, "He's been to the old country and *knows* something." Just as if any physician, though he may have been out of school for many years, does not, or may not, know of all the curative agencies of demonstrated merit!

Would a medical journal fail to keep its readers posted concerning any new discovery in medicine, or helpful appliance that promises real good to the profession? Yet people speak of one doctor's superior knowledge of the best treatment of a particular disease as if that doctor had access to some mysterious source of therapeutic knowledge unknown to other physicians. It is becoming less easy to work the "dangerous diagnosis" graft than formerly, for many people are learning that certain diseases must "run their course," and that there are no medicines that have specific curative effects on them.

There is another graft now that is taking the place of the one just mentioned, to some extent at least. In the hands of a fellow with lots of nerve and little conscience it is the greatest of them all. This is the graft of the smart young fellow direct from a post-graduate course in the clinics of some great surgeon.

He comes to town with a great flourish of trumpets. Of course, he observes the ethics of the profession! The long accounts of his superior education and unusual experience with operative surgery are only legitimate items of news for the local papers. Certainly! It is only right that such an unusual doctor should have so much attention.

There is no "starving time" for him. No weary wait of years for patients to come. At one bound he leaps into fame and fortune by performing "big operations" right and left, when before his coming such cases were only occasionally found, and then taken to surgeons of known ability and experience. The reputable physician respects surgery, and would respect the bright young fellow fresh from contact with the latest approved methods who has nerve to undertake the responsibility of a dangerous operation when such an operation is really indicated. But when it comes to mutilating the human body by cutting away an appendix or an ovary because it is known that to remove them when neither they nor the victim are much diseased is a comparatively safe and very *quick* way to get a big reputation—that is the limit of quackery. And no wonder such a man is so cordially hated by his brethren. He not always hated because he mutilates humanity so much, as because his spectacular graft in surgery is sure to be taken as proof conclusive that he is superior in all other departments of therapeutics.

And it puzzles observing laymen sometimes to know why all the successful (?) operations are considered such desirable items of news, while the cases that are not flattering in their outcome pass unmentioned.

I find most complete corroboration of my contention in the president's address, delivered before the Western Surgical and Gynecological Association at St. Louis, in 1907, by Charles W. Oviatt, M.D. This address was published in the *Journal of the American Medical Association*, and I herewith reprint it in part:

"The ambitious medical student does not usually get far into college work before he aspires to become a surgeon. He sees in the surgical clinics more definite and striking results than are discernible in other branches. Without being able to judge of his own relative fitness or whether he possesses the special aptitude so essential to success, he decides to become a surgeon. There will always be room for the young surgeon who, fitted by nature for the work, takes the time and opportunity to properly prepare himself. There is more good surgery being done to-day than ever before, and there are more good surgeons being educated to do the work. If, however, the surgeon of the future is to hold the high and honorable position our leaders have held in the past, there must be some standard of qualification established that shall protect the people against incompetency and dishonesty in surgeons.

"That there is much that passes under the name of surgery being done by ill-trained, incompetent men, will not be denied. What standard, then, should be established, and what requirement should be made before one should be permitted to do surgery? In his address as chairman of the Section on Surgery and Anatomy of the American Medical Association, at the Portland (1905) meeting, Dr. Maurice H. Richardson deals with this subject in such a forceful, clear-cut way, that I take the liberty to quote him at some length:

"'The burden of the following remarks is that those only should practice surgery who by education in the laboratory, in the dissecting-room, by the bedside, and at the operating-table, are qualified, first, to make reasonably correct deductions from subjective and objective signs; secondly, to give sound advice for or against operations; thirdly, to perform operations skillfully and quickly, and, fourthly, to conduct wisely the after-treatment.

"'The task before me is a serious criticism of what is going on in every community. I do not single out any community or any man. There is in my mind no doubt whatever that surgery is being practiced by those who are incompetent to practice it—by those whose education is imperfect, who lack natural aptitude, whose environment is such that they never can gain that personal experience which alone will really fit them for what surgery means to-day. They are unable to make correct deductions from histories; to predict probable events; to perform operations skillfully, or to manage after-treatment.

"'All surgeons are liable to error, not only in diagnosis, but in the performance of operations based on diagnosis. Such errors must always be expected and included in the contingencies of the practice of medicine and surgery. Doubtless many of my hearers can recall cases of their own in which useless—or worse than useless—operations have been performed. If, however, serious operations are in the hands of men of large experience, such errors will be reduced to a minimum.

"'Many physicians send patients for diagnosis and opinion as to the advisability of operation without telling the consultant that they themselves are to perform the operation. The diagnosis is made and the operation perhaps recommended, when it appears that the operation is to be in incompetent hands. His advice should be conditional that it be carried out only by the competent. Many operations, like the removal of the vermiform appendix in the period of health, the removal of fibroids which are not seriously offending, the removal of gall-stones that are not causing symptoms, are operations of choice rather than of necessity; they are operations which should never be advised unless they are to be performed by men of the greatest skill. Furthermore, many emergency operations, such as the removal of an inflamed appendix and other operations for lesions which are not necessarily fatal—should be forbidden and the patient left to the chances of spontaneous recovery, if the operation proposed is to be performed by an incompetent.

"'And is not the surgeon, appreciating his own unfitness in spite of years of devotion, in the position to condemn those who lightly take up such burdens without preparation and too often without conscience?

"'In view of these facts, who should perform surgery? How shall the surgeon be best fitted for these grave duties? As a matter of right and wrong, who shall, in the opinion of the medical profession, advise and perform these responsible acts and who shall not? Surgical operations should be performed only by those who are educated for that special purpose.

"'I have no hesitation in saying that the proper fitting of a man for surgical practice requires a much longer experience as a student and assistant than the most exacting schools demand. A man should serve four, five or six years as assistant to an active surgeon. During this period of preparation, as it were, as much time as possible should be given to observing the work of the masters of surgery throughout the world.'

"While Dr. Richardson's ideal may seem almost utopian, there being so wide a difference between the standard he would erect and the one generally established, we must all agree that however impossible of attainment under present conditions, such an ideal is none too high and its future realization not too much to hope for.

"While there is being done enough poor surgery that is honest and well intended, there is much being done that is useless, conscienceless, and done for purely commercial ends. This is truly a disagreeable and painful topic and one that I would gladly pass by, did I not feel that its importance demands some word of condemnation coming through such representative surgical organizations as this.

"The spirit of graft that has pervaded our ranks, especially here in the West, is doing much to lower the standard and undermine the morals and ethics of the profession. When fee-splitting and the paying of commissions for surgical work began to be heard of something like a decade ago, it seemed so palpably dishonest and wrong that it was believed that it would soon die out, or be at least confined to the few in whom the inherited commercial instinct was so strong that they could not get away from it. But it did not die; on the other hand, it has grown and flourished.

"In looking for an explanation for the existence of this evil, I think several factors must be taken into account, among them being certain changes in our social and economic conditions. This is an age of commercialism. We are known to the world as a nation of "dollar chasers," where nearly everything that should contribute to right living is sacrificed to the Moloch of money. The mad rush for wealth which has characterized the business world, has in a way induced some medical men, whether rightfully or wrongfully, to adopt the same measures in self-protection. The patient or his friends too often insist on measuring the value of our services with a commercial yard-stick, the fee to be paid being the chief consideration. In this way the public must come in for its share of responsibility for existing conditions. So long as there are people who care so little who operates on them, just so long will there be cheap surgeons, cheap in every respect, to supply the demand. The demand for better physicians and surgeons must come in part from those who employ their services.

"Another source of the graft evil is the existence of low-grade, irregular and stock-company medical schools. In many of these schools the entrance requirements are not in evidence outside of their catalogues. With no standard of character or ethics, these schools turn out men who have gotten the little learning they possess in the very atmosphere of graft. The existence of these schools seems less excusable when we consider that our leading medical colleges rank with the best in the world and are ample for the needs of all who should enter the profession. Their constant aim is to still further elevate the standard and to admit as students only those who give unmistakable evidence of being morally and intellectually fit to become members of the profession.

"Enough men of character, however, are entering the field through these better schools to ensure the upholding of those lofty ideals that have characterized the profession in the past and which are essential to our continued progress. I think, therefore, that we may take a hopeful view of the future. The demand for better prepared physicians will eventually close many avenues that are now open to students, greatly to the benefit of all. With the curtailing of the number of students and a less fierce competition which this will bring, there will be less temptation, less necessity, if you will, on the part of general practitioners to ask for a division of fees. He will come to see that honest dealing on his part with the patient requiring special skill will in the long run be the best policy. He will make a just, open charge for the services he has rendered and not attempt to collect a surreptitious fee through a dishonest surgeon for services he has not rendered and could not render. Then, too, there will be less inducement and less opportunity for incompetent and conscienceless men to disgrace the art of surgery.

"The public mind is becoming especially active just at this time in combating graft in all forms, and is ready to aid in its destruction. The intelligent portion of the laity is becoming alive to the patent medicine evil. It is only a question of time when the people will demand that the secular papers which go into our homes shall not contain the vile, disgusting and suggestive quack advertisements that are found to-day. A campaign of reform is being instituted against dishonest politicians, financiers, railroad and insurance magnates, showing that their methods will be no longer tolerated. The moral standards set for professional men and men in public life are going to be higher in the future, and with the limelight of public opinion turned on the medical and surgical grafter, the evil will cease to exist. Hand in hand with this reform let us hope that there will come to be established a legal and moral standard of qualification for those who assume to do surgery.

"I feel sure that it is the wish of every member of this association to do everything possible to hasten the coming of this day and to aid in the uplifting of the art of surgery. Our individual effort in this direction must lie largely through the influence we exert over those who seek our advice before beginning the study of medicine, and over those who, having entered the work, are to follow in our immediate footsteps. To the young man who seeks our counsel as to the advisability of commencing the study of medicine, it is our duty to make a plain statement of what would be expected of him, of the cost in time and money, and an estimate of what he might reasonably expect as a reward for a life devoted to ceaseless study, toil and responsibility. If, from our knowledge of the character, attainments and qualifications of the young man we feel that at best he could make but a modicum of success in the work, we should endeavor to divert his ambition into some other channel.

"We should advise the 'expectant surgeon' in his preparation to follow as nearly as possible the line of study suggested by Richardson. Then I would add the advice of Senn, viz: 'To do general practice for several years, return to laboratory work and surgical anatomy, attend the clinics of different operators, and never cease to be a physician. If this advice is followed there will be less unnecessary operating done in the future than has been the case in the past.' The young man who enters special work without having had experience as a general practitioner, is seriously handicapped. In this age, when we have so frequently to deal with the so-called border-line cases, it is especially well never to cease being a physician.

"We would next have the young man assure himself that he is the possessor of a well-developed, healthy, working 'surgical conscience.' No matter how well qualified he may be, his enthusiasm in the earlier years of his work will lead him to do operations that he would refrain from in later life. This will be especially true of malignant disease. He knows that early and thorough radical measures alone hold out hope, and only by repeated unsuccessful efforts will he learn to temper his ambition by the judgment that comes of experience. Pirogoff, the noted surgeon, suffered from a malignant growth. Billroth refused to operate or advise operation. In writing to another surgeon friend he said: 'I am not the bold operator whom you knew years ago in Zurich. Before deciding on the necessity of an operation, I always propose to myself this question: Would you permit such an operation as you intend performing on your patient to be done on yourself? Years and experience bring in their train a certain degree of hesitancy.' This, coming from one who in his day was the most brilliant operator in the world, should be remembered by every surgeon, young and old."

Oh, surgery! Modern aseptic surgery! In the hands of the skilled, conscientious surgeon how great are thy powers for good to suffering humanity! In the hands of shysters "what crimes are committed in thy name!"

With his own school full of shysters and incompetents, and grafters of "new schools" and "systems" to compete with on every hand, the conscientious physician seems to be "between the devil and the deep sea!"

With quacks to the right of him, quacks to the left of him, quacks in front of him, all volleying and thundering with their literature to prove that the old schools, and all schools other than theirs, are frauds, impostors and poisoners, about all that is left for the layman to do when sick is to take to the woods.

PART TWO
OSTEOPATHY

CHAPTER VII.

SOME DEFINITIONS AND HISTORIES.

Romantic Story of Osteopathy's Origin—An Asthma Cure—
Headache Cured by Plowlines—Log Rolling to Relieve
Dysentery—Osteopathy is Drugless Healing—Osteopathy is
Manual Treatment—Liberty of Blood, Nerves and Arteries—
Perfect Skeletal Alignment and Tonic, Ligamentous, Muscular
and Facial Relaxation—Andrew T. Still in 1874—Kirksville,
Mo., as a Mecca—American School of Osteopathy—The
Promised Golden Stream of Prosperity—Shams and Pretenses—
The "Mossbacks"—"Who's Who in Osteopathy."

The story of the origin of Osteopathy is romantic enough to
appeal to the fancy of impressionists. It is almost as romantic as
the finding of the mysterious stones by the immortal Joe Smith.
In this story is embodied the life history of an old-time doctor
and pioneer hero in his restless migrations about the frontiers of
Kansas and Missouri. His thrilling experiences in the days of
border wars and through the Civil War are narrated, and how the
germ of the idea of the true cause and cure of disease was planted
in his mind by the remark of a comrade as the two lay concealed
in a thicket for days to escape border ruffians. Then, later, how
the almost simultaneous death of two or three beloved children,
whom all his medical learning and that of other doctors he had
summoned had been powerless to save, had caused him to
renounce forever the belief that drugs could cure disease. He
believed Nature had a true system, and for this he began a patient
search. He wandered here and there, almost in the condition of

the religious reformers of old, who "wandered up and down clad in sheep-skins and goat-hides, of whom the world was not worthy." In the name of suffering humanity he desecrated the grave of poor Lo, that he might read from his red bones some clue to the secret.

One Osteopathic journal claims to tell authentically how Still was led to the discovery of the "great truth." It states that by accidentally curing a case of asthma by "fooling with the bones of the chest," he was led to the belief that bones out of normal position cause disease.

Still himself tells a rather different story in a popular magazine posing of late years as a public educator in matters of therapeutics. In this magazine Still tells how he discovered the principles of Osteopathy by curing a terrible headache resting the back of his neck across a swing made of his father's plowlines, and next by writhing on his back across a log to relieve the pain of dysentery. Accidentally the "lesion" was corrected, or the proper center "inhibited," and his headache and flux immediately cured.

You can take your choice of these various versions of the wonderful discovery.

Ever since Osteopathy began to attract attention, and people began to inquire "What is it?" its leading promoters have vied with each other in trying to construct a good definition for their "great new science."

Here are some of the definitions:

"Osteopathy is the science of drugless healing." For a genuine "lesion" Osteopath that would not do at all. It is too broad and gives too much scope to the physicians who would do more than "pull bones."

"Osteopathy is practical anatomy and physiology skillfully and scientifically applied as *manual* treatment of disease." That definition suits better, because of the "manual treatment." If you are a true Osteopath you must do it *all* with your hands. It will not do to use any mechanical appliances, for if you do you cannot keep up the impression that you are "handling the body with the skilled touch of a master who knows every part of his machine."

"The human body is a machine run by the unseen force called life, and that it may run harmoniously it is necessary that there be liberty of blood, nerves, and arteries from the generating point to destination." This definition may be impressive to the popular mind, but, upon analysis, we wonder if any other string of big words might not have had the same effect. "Liberty of blood" is a proposition even a stupid medical man must admit. Of course, there must be free circulation of blood, and massage, or hot and cold applications, or exercise, or anything that will stimulate circulation, is rational. But when "liberty of blood" is mentioned, what is meant by "liberty of arteries"?

"Osteopathy seeks to obtain perfect skeletal alignment and tonic ligamentous, muscular and facial relaxation." Some Osteopaths and other therapeutic reformers (?) have contended that medical men purposely used "big words" and Latin names to confound the laity. What must we think of the one just given as a popular definition?

A good many Osteopaths are becoming disgusted with the big words, technical terms and "high-sounding nothings" used by so many Osteopathic writers. The limit of this was never reached, however, until an A.B., Ph.D., D.O. wrote an article to elucidate Osteopathy for the general public in an American encyclopedia. It takes scholarly wisdom to simplify great truths and bring them to the comprehension of ordinary minds. If writers for the medical profession want a lesson in the art of simplifying and popularizing therapeutic science, they should study this article on Osteopathy in the encyclopedia.

A brief history of Osteopathy is perhaps in place. The following summary is taken from leading Osteopathic journals. As to the personality and motives of its founders I know but little; of the motives of its leading promoters a candid public must be the judge. But judgment should be withheld until all the truth is known.

The principles of Osteopathy were discovered by Dr. Andrew T. Still in 1874. He was at that time a physician of the old school practicing in Kansas. His father, brothers and uncles were all medical practitioners. He was at one time scout surgeon under General Fremont. During the Civil War he was surgeon in the Union army in a volunteer corps. It was during the war that he began to lose faith in drugs, and to search for something natural in combating disease.

Then began a long struggle with poverty and abuse. He was obstructed by his profession and ridiculed by his friends. Fifteen years after the discovery of Osteopathy found Dr. Still located in the little town of Kirksville, Mo., where he had gradually attracted a following who had implicit faith in his power to heal by what to them seemed mysterious movements.

His fame spread beyond the town, and chronic sufferers began to turn toward Kirksville as a Mecca of healing. Others began to desire Still's healing powers. In 1892 the American School of Osteopathy was founded, which from a small beginning has grown until the present buildings and equipment cost more than $100,000. Hundreds of students are graduated yearly from this school, and large, well-equipped schools have been founded in Des Moines, Philadelphia, Boston and California, with a number of schools of greater or less magnitude scattered in other parts of the country. More than four thousand Osteopaths were in the field in 1907, and this number is being augmented every year by a larger number of physicians than are graduated from Homeopathic colleges, according to Osteopathic reports.

About thirty-five States have given Osteopathy more or less favorable legal recognition.

The discussion of the subject of Osteopathy is of very grave importance. Important to practitioners of the old schools of medicine for reasons I shall give further on, and of vital importance to the thousands of men and women who have chosen Osteopathy as their life work. It is even of greater importance in another sense to the people who are called upon to decide which system is right, and which school they ought to rely upon when their lives are at stake.

I shall try to speak advisedly and conservatively, as I wish to do no one injustice. I should be sorry indeed to speak a word that might hinder the cause of truth and progress. I started out to tell of all that prevents the sway of truth and honesty in therapeutics. I should come far short of telling all if I omitted the inconsistencies of this "new science" of healing that dares to assume the responsibility for human life, and makes bold to charge that time-tried systems, with their tens of thousands of practitioners, are wrong, and that the right remedy, or the best remedy for disease has been unknown through all these years until the coming of Osteopathy. And further dares to make the still more serious charge that since the truth has been brought to light, the majority of medical men are so blinded by prejudice or ignorance that they *will* not see.

This is not the first time I have spoken about inconsistencies in the practice of Osteopathy. I saw so much of it in a leading Osteopathic college that when I had finished I could not conscientiously proclaim myself as an exponent of a "complete and well-rounded system of healing, adequate for every emergency," as Osteopathy is heralded to be by the journals published for "Osteopathic physicians" to scatter broadcast among the people. I practiced Osteopathy for three years, but only as an Osteopathic specialist. I never during that time accepted responsibility for human life when I did not feel sure that I could do as much for the case as any other might do with other means or some other system.

Because I practiced as a specialist and would not claim that Osteopathy would cure everything that any other means might cure, I have never been called a good disciple of the new science by my brethren. I would not practice as a grafter, find bones dislocated and "subluxated," and tell people that they must take two or three months' treatment at twenty-five dollars per month, to have one or two "subluxations" corrected. In consequence I was never overwhelmed by the golden stream of prosperity the literature that made me a convert had assured me would be forthcoming to all "Osteopathic physicians" of even ordinary ability.

As I said, this is not the first time I have spoken of the inconsistencies of Osteopathy. While yet in active practice I became so disgusted with some of the shams and pretences that I wrote a long letter to the editor of an Osteopathic journal published for the good of the profession. This editor, a bright and capable man, wrote me a nice letter in reply, in which he agreed with me about quackery and incompetency in our profession. He did not publish the letter I wrote, or express his honest sentiments, as I had hoped he might. If what I wrote to that editor was the truth, as he acknowledged in private, it is time the public knew something of it. I believe, also, that many of the large number of Osteopaths who have been discouraged or disgusted, and quit the practice, will approve what I am writing. There is another class of Osteopathic practitioners who, I believe, will welcome the truth I have to tell. This consists of the large number of men and women who are practicing Osteopathy as standing for all that makes up rational physio-therapy.

Speaking of those who have quit the practice of Osteopathy, I will say that they are known by the Osteopathic faculties to be a large and growing number. Yet Osteopathic literature sent to prospective students tells of the small per cent. of those who take the course who fail. It may not be known how many fail, but it is known that many have quit.

A journey half across one of our Western States disclosed one Osteopath in the meat business, one in the real estate business, one clerking in a store, and two, a blind man and his wife, fairly prosperous Osteopathic physicians. This was along one short line of railroad, and there is no reason why it may not be taken as a sample of the percentage of those who have quit in the entire country.

I heard three years ago from a bright young man who graduated with honors, started out with luxurious office rooms in a flourishing city, and was pointed to as an example of the prosperity that comes to the Osteopath from the very start. When I heard from him last he was advance bill-poster for a cheap show. Another bright classmate was carrying a chain for surveyors in California.

I received an Osteopathic journal recently containing a list of names, about eight hundred of them, of "mossbacks," as we were politely called. I say "we," for my name was on the list. The journal said these were the names of Osteopaths whose addresses were lost and no communication could be had with them. They were wanted badly, it seemed. Just for what, aside from the annual fee to the American Osteopathic Association, was not clear.

I do know what the silence of a good many of them meant. They have quit, and do not care to read the abuse that some of the

Osteopathic journals are continually heaping upon those who do not keep their names on the "Who's Who in Osteopathy" list.

There is a large percentage of failures in other professions, and it is not strange that there should be some in Osteopathy. But when Osteopathic journals dwell upon the large chances of success and prosperity for those who choose Osteopathy as a profession, those who might become students should know the other side.

CHAPTER VIII.

THE OSTEOPATHIC PROPAGANDA.

Wonderful Growth Claimed to Prove Merit—Osteopathy is Rational Physio-Therapy—Growth is in Exact Proportion to Advertising Received—Booklets and Journals for Gratuitous Distribution—Osteopathy Languishes or Flourishes by Patent Medicine Devices—Circular Letter from Secretary of American Osteopathic Association—Boosts by Governors and Senators—The Especial Protege of Authors—Mark Twain—Opie Reed—Emerson Hough—Sam Jones—The Orificial Surgeon—The M.D. Seeking Job as "Professor"—The Lure of "Honored Doctor" with "Big Income"—No Competition.

But what about Osteopathy? Why has it had such a wonderful growth in popularity? Why have nearly four thousand men and women, most of them intelligent and some of them educated, espoused it as a profession to follow as a life work? These are questions I shall now try to answer.

Osteopathic promoters and enthusiasts claim that the wonderful growth and popularity of Osteopathy prove beyond question its merits as a healing system. I have already dealt at length with reasons why intelligent people are so ready to fall victims to new systems of healing. The "perfect adjustment," "perfect functioning" theory of Osteopathy is especially attractive to people made ripe for some "drugless healing" system by causes already mentioned. When Osteopathy is practiced as a combination of all manipulations and other natural aids to the inherent recuperative powers of the body, it will appeal to reason in such a way and bring such good results as to make and keep friends.

I am fully persuaded, and I believe the facts when presented will establish it, that it is the physio-therapy in Osteopathy that wins and holds the favor of intelligent people. But Osteopathy in its own name, taught as "a well-rounded system of healing adequate for every emergency," has grown and spread largely as a "patent medicine" flourishes, *i. e.*, in exact proportion to the advertising it has received. I would not presume to make this statement as merely my opinion. The question at issue is too important to be treated as a matter of opinion. I will present facts, and let my readers settle the point in their own minds.

Every week I get booklets or "sample copies" of journals heralding the wonderful curative powers of Osteopathy. These are published not as journals for professional reading, but to be sold to the practitioners by the hundreds or thousands, to be given to their patients for distribution by these patients to their friends. The publishers of these "boosters" say, and present testimonials to prove it, that Osteopaths find their practice languishes or flourishes just in proportion to the numbers of these journals and booklets they keep circulating in their communities. Here is a sample testimonial I received some time since on a postal card:

"Gentlemen: Since using your journals more patients have come to me than I could treat, many of them coming from neighboring towns. Quite a number have had to go home without being treated, leaving their names so that they could be notified later, as I can get to them. Your booklets bring them O. K."

The boast is often made that Osteopathy is growing in spite of bitter opposition and persecution, and is doing it on its merits—doing it because "Truth is mighty and will prevail." At one time I honestly believed this to be true, but I have been convinced by highest Osteopathic authority that it is not true. As some of that proof here is an extract from a circular letter from the secretary of the American Osteopathic Association:

"Now, Doctor, we feel that you have the success of Osteopathy at heart, and if you realize the activity and complete organization of the American Medical Association and their efforts to curb our limitations, and do not become a member of this Association, which stands opposed to the efforts of the big monopoly, we must believe that you are not familiar with the earnestness of the A. O. A. and its efforts. We must work in harmonious accord and with an organized purpose. *When we rest on our oars the death knell begins to sound.* Can you not see that unless you co-operate with your fellow-practitioners in this national effort you are *sounding your own limitations?*"

This from the *secretary* of the American Osteopathic Association, when we have boasted of superior equipment for intelligent physicians. Incidentally we pause to make excuse for the expressions: "Curbing our limitations" and "sounding your own limitations."

But does the idea that when we quit working as an organized body *"our death knell begins to sound,"* indicate that Osteopathic leaders are content to trust the future of Osteopathy to its merits?

If Osteopathic promoters do not feel that the life of their science depends on boosting, what did the secretary of the A.O.A. mean when he said, "Upon the success of these efforts depends the weal or woe of Osteopathy as an independent system"? If truth always grows under persecution, how can the American Medical Association kill Osteopathy when it is so well known by the people?

Nearly four thousand Osteopaths are scattered in thirty-six States where they have some legal recognition, and they are treating thousands of invalids every day. If they are performing the wonderful cures Osteopathic journals tell of, why are we told that the welfare of the system depends upon the noise that is made and the boosting that is done?

Has it required advertising to keep people using anesthetics since it was demonstrated that they would prevent pain?

Has it required boosting to keep the people resorting to surgery since the benefits of modern operations have been proved?

Does it look as if Osteopathy has been standing or advancing on its merits? Does it not seem that Osteopathy, as a complete system, is mostly a *name*, and "lives, moves, and has its being" in boosting? It seems to have been about the best boosted fad ever fancied by a foolish people. Governors and senators have boosted for it. Osteopathic journals have published again and again the nice things a number of governors said when they signed the bills investing Osteopathy with the dignity of State authority.

A certain United States senator from Ohio has won more notoriety as a champion of Osteopathy than he has lasting fame as a statesman.

Osteopathy has been the especial protégé of authors. Mark Twain once went up to Albany and routed an army of medical lobbyists who were there to resist the passage of a bill favorable to Osteopathy. For this heroic deed Mark is better known to Osteopaths to-day than even for his renowned history of Huckleberry Finn. He is in danger of losing his reputation as a champion of the "under dog in the fight." Lately he has gone on the warpath again. This time to annihilate poor Mother Eddy and her fond delusion.

Opie Reed is a delightful writer while he sticks to the portrayal of droll Southern character. Ella Wheeler Wilcox is admirable for the beauty and boldness with which she portrays the passions and emotions of humanity. But they are both better known to Osteopaths for the bouquets they have tossed at Osteopathy than for their profound human philosophy that used to be promulgated by the *Chicago American.*

Emerson Hough gave a little free advertising in his "Heart's Desire." There may have been "method in his madness," for that Osteopathic horse doctoring scene no doubt sold many a book for the author.

Sam Jones also helped along with some of his striking originality. Sam said, "There is as much difference between Osteopathy and massage as between playing a piano and currying a horse." The idea of comparing the Osteopath's manipulations of the human body to the skilled touch of the pianist upon his instrument was especially pleasing to Osteopaths. However, Sam displayed about the same comprehension of his subject that preachers usually exhibit who try to say nice things about the doctors when they get their doctoring gratis or at reduced rates.

These champions of Osteopathy no doubt mean well. They can be excused on the ground that they got out of place to aid in the cause of "struggling truth." But what shall we say of medical men, some of them of reputation and great influence, who uphold and champion new systems under such conditions that it is questionable whether they do it from principle or policy?

Osteopathic journals have made much of an article written by a famous "orificial surgeon." The article appears on the first page of a leading Osteopath journal, and is headed, "An Expert Opinion on Osteopathy." Among the many good things he says of the "new science" is this: "The full benefit of a single sitting can be secured in from three to ten minutes instead of an hour or more, as required by massage." I shall discuss the time of an average Osteopathic treatment further on, but I should like to see how long this brother would hold his practice if he were an Osteopath and treated from three to ten minutes.

He also says that "Osteopathy is so beneficial to cases of insanity that it seems quite probable that this large class of terrible sufferers may be almost emancipated from their hell." I shall also say more further on of what I know of Osteopathy's record as an insanity cure. There is this significant thing in connection with this noted specialist's boost for Osteopathy. The journal printing this article comments on it in another number; tells what a great man the specialist is, and incidentally lets Osteopaths know that if any of them want to add a knowledge of "orificial surgery" to their "complete science," this doctor is the man from whom to get it, as he is the "great and only" in his specialty, and is big and broad enough to appreciate Osteopathy.

The most despicable booster of any new system of therapeutics is the physician who becomes its champion to get a job as "professor" in one of its colleges. Of course it is a strong temptation to a medical man who has never made much of a reputation in his own profession.

You may ask, "Have there been many such medical men?" Consult the faculty rolls of the colleges of these new sciences, and you will be surprised, no doubt, to find how many put M.D. after their names. Why are they there? Some of these were honest converts to the system, perhaps. Some wanted the honor of being "Professor Doctor," maybe, and some may have been lured by the same bait that attracts so many students into Osteopathic colleges. That is, the positive assurance of "plenty of easy money" in it.

One who has studied the real situation in an effort to learn why Osteopathy has grown so fast as a profession, can hardly miss the conclusion that advertising keeps the grist of students pouring into Osteopathic mills. There is scarcely a corner of the United States that their seductive literature does not reach. Practitioners in the field are continually reminded by the schools from which they graduated that their alma mater looks largely to their solicitations to keep up the supply of recruits.

Their advertising, the tales of wonderful cures and big money made, appeal to all classes. It seems that none are too scholarly and none too ignorant to become infatuated with the idea of becoming an "honored doctor" with a "big income." College professors and preachers have been lured from comfortable positions to become Osteopaths. Shrewd traveling men, seduced by the picture of a permanent home, have left the road to become Osteopathic physicians and be "rich and honored."

Other classes come also. To me, when a student of Osteopathy, it was pathetic and almost tragic to observe the crowds of men and women who had been seduced from spheres of drudging usefulness, such as clerking, teaching, barbering, etc., to become money-making doctors. In their old callings they had lost all hope of gratifying ambition for fame and fortune, but were making an honest living. The rosy pictures of honor, fame and twenty dollars per day, that the numerous Osteopathic circulars and journals painted, were not to be withstood.

These circulars told them that the fields into which they might go and reap that $20 per day were unlimited. They said: "There are dozens of ministers ready to occupy each vacant pulpit, and as many applicants for each vacancy in the schools. Each hamlet has four or five doctors, where it can support but one. The legal profession is filled to the starving point. Young licentiates in the older professions all have to pass through a starving time. Not so in Osteopathy. There is no competition." The picture was a rosy dream of triumphant success! When they had mastered the great science and become "Doctors of Osteopathy," the world was waiting with open arms and pocketbooks to receive them.

CHAPTER IX.

THEORY AND PRACTICE OF OSTEOPATHY.

Infallible, Touch-the-Button System that Always Cured—Indefinite Movements and Manipulations—Wealth of Undeveloped Scientific Facts—Osteopaths Taking M.D. Course—The Standpatter and the Drifter—The "Lesionist"—"Bone Setting"—"Inhibiting a Center"—Chiropractics—"Finest Anatomists in the World"—How to Cure Torticollis, Goitre and Enteric Troubles—A Successful Osteopath—Timid Old Maids—Osteopathic Philanthropy.

How desperately those students worked. Many of them were men and women with gray heads, who had found themselves stranded at a time of life when they should have been able to retire on a competency. They had staked their little all on this last venture, and what was before them if they should fail heaven only knew. How eagerly they looked forward to the time when they should have struggled through the lessons in anatomy, chemistry, physiology, symptomatology and all the rest, and should be ready to receive the wonderful principles of Osteopathy they were to apply in performing the miraculous cures that were to make them wealthy and famous. Need I tell the physician who was a conscientious student of anatomy in his school days, that there was disappointment when the time came to enter the class in "theory and practice" of Osteopathy?

There had been vague ideas of a systematized, infallible, touch-the-button system that *always* cured. Instead, we were instructed in a lot of indefinite movements and manipulations that somehow left us speculating as to just how much of it all was done for effect.

We had heard so often that Osteopathy was a complete satisfying science *that did things specifically!* Now it began to dawn upon us that there was indeed a "wealth of undeveloped scientific facts" in Osteopathy, as those glittering circulars had said when they thought to attract young men ambitious for original research. They had said, "Much yet remains to be discovered." Some of us wondered if the "undeveloped" and "undiscovered" scientific facts were not the main constituents of the "science."

The students expected something exact and tangible, and how eagerly they grasped at anything in the way of bringing quick results in curing the sick.

If Osteopathy is so complete, why did so many students, after they had received everything the learned (?) professors had to impart, procure Juettner's "Modern Physio-Therapy" and Ling's "Manual Therapy" and Rosse's "Cures Without Drugs" and Kellogg's work on "Hydrotherapy"? They felt that they needed all they could get.

It was customary for the students to begin "treating" after they had been in school a few months, and medical men will hardly be surprised to know that they worked with more faith in their healing powers and performed more wonderful (?) cures in their freshman year than they ever did afterward.

I have in mind a student, one of the brightest I ever met, who read a cheap book on Osteopathic practice, went into a community where he was unknown, and practiced as an Osteopathic physician. In a few months he had made enough money to pay his way through an Osteopathic college, which he entered professing to believe that Osteopathy would cure all the ills flesh is heir to, but which he left two years later to take a medical course. He secured his D.O. degree, but I notice that it is his M.D. degree he flourishes with pride.

Can students be blamed for getting a little weak in faith when men who told them that the great principles of Osteopathy were sufficient to cure *everything*, have been known to backslide so far as to go and take medical courses themselves?

How do you suppose it affects students of an Osteopathic college to read in a representative journal that the secretary of their school, and the greatest of all its boosters, calls medical men into his own family when there is sickness in it?

There are many men and women practicing to-day who try to be honest and conscientious, and by using all the good in Osteopathy, massage, Swedish movements, hydrotherapy, and all the rest of the adjuncts of physio-therapy, do a great deal of good. The practitioner who does use these agencies, however, is denounced by the stand-patters as a "drifter." They say he is not a true Osteopath, but a mongrel who is belittling the great science. That circular letter from the secretary of the American Osteopathic Association said that one of the greatest needs of organization was to preserve Osteopathy in its primal purity as it came from its founder, A. T. Still.

If our medical brethren and the laity could read some of the acrimonious discussions on the question of using adjuncts, they would certainly be impressed with the exactness (?) of Osteopathic science.

There is one idea of Osteopathy that even the popular mind has grasped, and that is that it is essentially finding "lesions" and correcting them. Yet the question has been very prominent and pertinent among Osteopaths: "Are you a lesion Osteopath?" Think of it, gentlemen, asking an Osteopath if he is a "lesionist"! Yet there are plenty of Osteopaths who are stupid enough (or honest enough) not to be able to find bones "subluxed" every time they look at a patient. Practitioners who really want to do their patrons good will use adjuncts even if they are denounced by the stand-patters.

I believe every conscientious Osteopath must sometimes feel that it is safer to use rational remedies than to rely on "bone setting," or "inhibiting a center," but for the grafter it is not so spectacular and involves more hard work.

The stand-patters of the American Osteopathic Association have not eliminated all trouble when they get Osteopaths to stick to the "bone setting, inhibiting" idea. The chiropractic man threatens to steal their thunder here. The Chiropractor has found that when it comes to using mysterious maneuvers and manipulations as bases for mind cure, one thing is about as good as another, except that the more mysterious a thing looks the better it works. So the Chiropractor simply gives his healing "thrusts" or his wonderful "adjustments," touches the buttons along the spine as it were, when—presto! disease has flown before his healing touch and blessed health has come to reign instead!

The Osteopath denounces the Chiropractor as a brazen fraud who has stolen all that is good in Chiropractics (if there *is* anything good) from Osteopathy. But Chiropractics follows so closely what the "old liner" calls the true theory of Osteopathy that, between him and the drifter who gives an hour of crude massage, or uses the forbidden accessories, the true Osteopath has a hard time maintaining the dignity (?) of Osteopathy and keeping its practitioners from drifting.

Some of the most ardent supporters of true Osteopathy I have ever known have drifted entirely away from it. After practicing two or three years, abusing medicine and medical men all the time, and proclaiming to the people continually that they had in Osteopathy all that a sick world could ever need, it is suddenly learned that the "Osteopath is gone." He has "silently folded his tent and stolen away," and where has he gone? He has gone to a medical college to study that same medicine he has so industriously abused while he was gathering in the shekels as an Osteopath. Going to learn and practice the science he has so persistently denounced as a fraud and a curse to humanity.

The intelligent, conscientious Osteopath who dares to brave the scorn of the stand-patter and use all the legitimate adjuncts of Osteopathy found in physio-therapy, may do a great deal of good as a physician. I have found many physicians willing to acknowledge this, and even recommend the services of such an Osteopath when physio-therapy was indicated.

When a physician, however, meets a fellow who claims to have in his Osteopathy a wonderful system, complete and all-sufficient to cope with any and all diseases, and that his system is founded on a knowledge of the relation and function of the various parts and organs of the body such as no other school of therapeutics has ever been able to discover, then he knows that he has met a man of the same mental and moral calibre as the shyster in his own school. He knows he has met a fellow who is exploiting a thing, that may be good in its way and place, as a graft. And he knows that this grafter gets his wonderful cures largely as any other quack gets his; the primary effects of his "scientific manipulations" are on the minds of those treated.

The intelligent physician knows that the Osteopath got his boastedly superior knowledge of anatomy mostly from the same text-books and same class of cadavers that other physicians had to master if they graduated from a reputable school. All that talk we have heard so much about the Osteopaths being the "finest anatomists in the world" sounds plausible, and is believed by the laity generally.

The quotation I gave above has been much used in Osteopathic literature as coming from an eminent medical man. What foundation is there for such a belief? The Osteopath *may* be a good anatomist. He has about the same opportunities to learn anatomy the medical student has. If he is a good and conscientious student he may consider his anatomy of more importance than does the medical student who is not expecting to do much surgery. If he is a natural shyster and shirk he can get through a course in Osteopathy and get his diploma, and this diploma may be about the only proof he could ever give that he is a "superior anatomist."

Great stress has always been laid by Osteopaths upon the amount of study and research done by their students on the cadaver. I want to give you some specimens of the learning of the man (an M.D.) who presided over the dissecting-room when I pursued my "profound research" on the "lateral half." This great man, whose superior knowledge of anatomy, I presume, induced by the wise management of the college to employ him as a demonstrator, in an article written for the organ of the school expresses himself thus:

"It is needless to say that the first impression of an M. D. would not be favorable to Osteopathy, because he has spent years fixing in his mind that if you had a bad case of torticollis not to touch it, but give a man morphine or something of the same character with an external blister or hot application and in a week or ten days he would be all right. In the meanwhile watch the patient's general health, relieve the induced constipation by suitable means and rearrange what he has disarranged in his treatment. On the other hand, let the Osteopath get hold of this patient, and with his *vast* and we might say *perfect* knowledge of anatomy, he at once, with no other tools than his hands, inhibits the nerves supplying the affected parts, and in five minutes the patient can freely move his head and shoulders, entirely relieved from pain. Would not the medical man be angry? Would he not feel like wiping off the earth with all the Osteopaths? Doctor, with your medical education a course in Osteopathy would teach you that it is not necessary to subject your patients to myxedema by removing the thyroid gland to cure goitre. You would not have to lie awake nights studying means to stop one of those troublesome bowel complaints in children, nor to insist upon the enforced diet in chronic diarrhea, and a thousand other things which are purely physiological and are not done by any magical presto change, but by methods which are perfectly rational if you will only listen long enough to have them explained to you. I will agree that at first impression all methods look alike to the medical man, but when explained by an intelligent teacher they will bring their just reward."

Gentlemen of the medical profession, study the above carefully— punctuation, composition, profound wisdom and all. Surely you did not read it when it was given to the world a few years ago, or you would all have been converted to Osteopathy then, and the medical profession left desolate. We have heard many bad things of medical men, but never (until we learned it from one who was big-brained enough to accept Osteopathy when its great truths dawned upon him) did we know that you are so dull of intellect that it takes you "years to fix in your minds that if you had a bad case of torticollis not to touch it but to give a man morphine."

And how pleased Osteopaths are to learn from this scholar that the Osteopath can "take hold" of a case of torticollis, "and with his vast and we might say perfect knowledge of anatomy" inhibit the nerves and have the man cured in five minutes. We were glad to learn this great truth from this learned ex-M.D., as we never should have known, otherwise, that Osteopathy is so potent.

I have had cases of torticollis in my practice, and thought I had done well if after a half hour of hard work massaging contracted muscles I had benefited the case.

And note the relevancy of these questions, "Would not the medical man be angry? Would he not feel like wiping off the earth all the Osteopaths?" Gentlemen, can you explain your exbrother's meaning here? Surely you are not all so hard-hearted that you would be angry because a poor wry-necked fellow had been cured in five minutes.

To be serious, I ask you to think of "the finest anatomists in the world" doing their "original research" work in the dissecting-room under the direction of a man of the scholarly attainments indicated by the composition and thought of the above article. Do you see now how Osteopaths get a "vast and perfect knowledge of anatomy"?

Do you suppose that the law of "the survival of the fittest" determines who continues in the practice of Osteopathy and succeeds? Is it true worth and scholarly ability that get a big reputation of success among medical men? I know, and many medical men know from competition with him (if they would admit that such a fellow may be a competitor), that the ignoramus who as a physician is the product of a diploma mill often has a bigger reputation and performs more wonderful cures (?) than the educated Osteopath who really mastered the prescribed course but is too conscientious to assume responsibility for human life when he is not sure that he can do all that might be done to save life.

I once met an Osteopath whose literary attainments had never reached the rudiments of an education. He had never really comprehended a single lesson of his entire course. He told me that he was then on a vacation to get much-needed rest. He had such a large practice that the physical labor of it was wearing him out. I knew of this fellow's qualifications, but I thought he might be one of those happy mortals who have the faculty of "doing things," even if they cannot learn the theory. To learn the secret of this fellow's success, if I could, I let him treat me. I had some contracted muscles that were irritating nerves and holding joints in tense condition, a typical case, if there are any, for an Osteopathic treatment. The fellow began his "treatment." I expected him to do some of that "expert Osteopathic diagnosing" that you have heard of, but he began in an aimless desultory way, worked almost an hour, found nothing specific, did nothing but give me a poor unsystematic massage. He was giving me a "popular treatment."

In many towns people have come to estimate the value of an Osteopathic treatment by its duration. People used to say to me, "You don't treat as long as Dr. ———, who was here before you," and say it in a way indicating that they were hardly satisfied they had gotten their money's worth. Some of them would say: "He treated me an hour for seventy-five cents." Does it seem funny to talk of adjusting lesions on one person for an hour at a time, three times a week?

My picture of incompetency and apparent success of incompetents, is not overdrawn. The other day I had a marked copy of a local paper from a town in California. It was a flattering write-up of an old classmate. The doctor's automobile was mentioned, and he had marked with a cross a fine auto shown in a picture of the city garage. This fellow had been considered by all the Simple Simon of the class, inferior in almost every attribute of true manliness, yet now he flourishes as one of those of our class to whose success the school can "point with pride."

It is interesting to read the long list of "changes of location" among Osteopaths, yet between the lines there is a sad story that may be read. How often I have followed these changes. First, "Doctor Blank has located in Philadelphia, with twenty-five patients for the first month and rapidly growing practice." A year or so after another item tells that "Doctor Blank has located in San Francisco with bright prospects." Then "Doctor Blank has returned to Missouri on account of his wife's health, and located in ———, where he has our best wishes for success." Their career reminds us of Goldsmith's lines:

"As the hare whom horn and hounds pursue
Pants to the place from whence at first he flew."

There has been many a tragic scene enacted upon the Osteopathic stage, but the curtain has not been raised for the public to behold them. How many timid old maids, after saving a few hundred dollars from wages received for teaching school, have been persuaded that they could learn Osteopathy while their shattered nerves were repaired and they were made young and beautiful once more by a course of treatment in the clinics of the school. Then they would be ready to go out to occupy a place of dignity and honor, and treat ten to thirty patients per month at twenty-five dollars per patient.

Gentlemen of the medical profession, from what you know of the aggressive spirit that it takes to succeed in professional life to-day (to say nothing of the physical strength required in the practice of Osteopathy), what per cent. of these timid old maids do you suppose have "panted to the place from whence at first they flew," after leaving their pitiful little savings with the benefactors of humanity who were devoting their splendid talents to the cause of Osteopathy?

If any one doubts that some Osteopathic schools are conducted from other than philanthropic motives, let him read what the *Osteopathic Physician* said of a new school founded in California. Of all the fraud, bare-faced shystering, and flagrant rascality ever exposed in any profession, the circumstances of the founding of this school, as depicted by the editor of the *Osteopathic Physician*, furnishes the most disgusting instance. Men to whom we had clung when the anchor of our faith in Osteopathy seemed about to drag were held up before us as sneaking, cringing, incompetent rascals, whose motives in founding the school were commercial in the worst sense. And how do you suppose Osteopaths out in the field of practice feel when they receive catalogues from the leading colleges that teach their system, and these catalogues tell of the superior education the colleges are equipped to give, and among the pictures of learned members of the faculty they recognize the faces of old schoolmates, with glasses, pointed beards and white ties, silk hats maybe, but the same old classmate of—sometimes not ordinary ability.

I spoke a moment ago of old maids being induced to believe that they would be made over in the clinics of an Osteopathic college. That was not an exaggeration. An Osteopathic journal before me says: "If it were generally known that Osteopathy has a wonderfully rejuvenating effect upon fading beauty, Osteopathic physicians would be overworked as beauty doctors."

Another journal says: "If the aged could know how many years might be added to their lives by Osteopathy, they would not hesitate to avail themselves of treatment."

A leading D. O. discusses consumption as treated Osteopathically, and closes his discussion with the statement in big letters: "CONSUMPTION CAN BE CURED."

Another Osteopathic doctor says the curse that was placed upon Mother Eve in connection with the propagation of the race has been removed by Osteopathy, and childbirth "positively painless" is a consummated fact.

The old made young! The homely made beautiful! The insane emancipated from their hell! Consumption cured! Childbirth robbed of its terrors! Asthma cured by moving a bone! What more in therapeutics is left to be desired? O grave, where is thy victory?

CHAPTER X.

OSTEOPATHY AS RELATED TO SOME OTHER FAKES.

Sure Shot Rheumatism Cure—Regular Practitioner's Discomfiture—Medicines Alone Failed to Cure Rheumatism—Osteopathy Relieves Rheumatic and Neuralgic Pains—"Move Things"—"Pop" Stray Cervical Vertebræ—Find Something Wrong and Put it Right—Terrible Neck-Wrenching, Bone-Twisting Ordeal.

A discussion of graft in connection with doctoring would not be complete if nothing were said about the traveling medicine faker. Every summer our towns are visited by smooth-tongued frauds who give free shows on the streets. They harangue the people by the hour with borrowed spiels, full of big medical terms, and usually full of abuse of regular practitioners, which local physicians must note with humiliation is too often received by people without resentment and often with applause.

Only last summer I was standing by while one of these grafters was making his spiel, and gathering dollars by the pocketful for a "sure shot" rheumatism cure. His was a *sure* cure, doubly guaranteed; no cure, money all refunded (if you could get it). A physician standing near laughed rather a mirthless laugh, and remarked that Barnum was right when he said, "The American people like to be humbugged." When the medical man left, a man who had just become the happy possessor of enough of the wonderful herb to make a quart of the rheumatism router, remarked: "He couldn't be a worse humbug than that old duffer. He doctored me for six weeks, and told me all the time that his medicine would cure me in a few days. I got worse all the time until I went to Dr. ———, who told me to use a sack of hot bran mash on my back, and I was able to get around in two days."

In this man's remarks there is an explanation of the reason the crowd laughed when they heard the quack abusing the regular practitioner, and of the reason the people handed their hard-earned dollars to the grafter at the rate of forty in ten minutes, by actual count. If all doctors were honest and told the people what all authorities have agreed upon about rheumatism, *i. e.,* that internal medication does it little good, and the main reliance must be on external application, traveling and patent medicine fakers who make a specialty of rheumatism cure would be "put out of business," and there would be eliminated one source of much loss of faith in medicine.

I learned by experience as an Osteopath that many people lose faith in medicine and in the honesty of physicians because of the failure of medicine to cure rheumatism where the physician had promised a cure. Patients afflicted with other diseases get well anyway, or the sexton puts them where they cannot tell people of the physician's failure to cure them. The rheumatic patient lives on, and talks on of "Doc's" failure to stop his rheumatic pains. All doctors know that rheumatism is the universal disease of our fickle climate. If it were not for rheumatic pains, and neuralgic pains that often come from nerves irritated by contracted muscles, the Osteopath in the average country town would get more lonesome than he does. People who are otherwise skeptical concerning the merits of Osteopathy will admit that it seems rational treatment for rheumatism.

Yet this is a disease that Osteopathy of the specific-adjustment, bone-setting, nerve-inhibiting brand has little beneficial effect upon. All the Osteopathic treatments I ever gave or saw given in cases of rheumatism that really did any good, were long, laborious massages. The medical man who as "professor" in an Osteopathic college said, "When the Osteopath with his *vast* knowledge of anatomy gets hold of a case of torticollis he inhibits the nerves and cures it in five minutes," was talking driveling rot.

I have seen some of the best Osteopaths treat wry-neck, and the work they did was to knead and stretch and pull, which by starting circulation and working out soreness, gradually relieved the patient. A hot application, by expanding tissues and stimulating circulation, would have had the same effect, perhaps more slowly manifested.

To call any Osteopathic treatment massage is always resented as an insult by the guardians of the science. What is the Osteopath doing, who rolls and twists and pulls and kneads for a full hour, if he isn't giving a massage treatment? Of course, it sounds more dignified, and perhaps helps to "preserve the purity of Osteopathy as a separate system," to call it "reducing subluxations," "correcting lesions," "inhibiting and stimulating" nerves. The treatment also acts better as a placebo to call it by these names.

As students we were taught that all Osteopathic movements were primarily to adjust something. Some of us worried for fear we wouldn't know when the adjusting was complete. We were told that all the movements we were taught to make were potent to "move things," so we worried again for fear we might move something in the wrong direction. We were assured, however, that since the tendency was always toward the normal, all we had to do was to agitate, stir things up a bit, and the thing out of place would find its place. How *specific!* How scientific!

We were told that when in the midst of our "agitation" we heard something "pop," we could be sure the thing out of place had gone back. When a student had so mastered the great bone-setting science as to be able to "pop" stray cervical vertebræ he was looked upon with envy by the fellows who had not joined the association for protection against suits for malpractice, and did not know just how much of an owl they could make of a man and not break his neck.

The fellow who lacked clairvoyant powers to locate straying things, and could not always find the "missing link" of the spine, could go through the prescribed motions just the same. If he could do it with sufficient facial contortions to indicate supreme physical exertion, and at the same time preserve the look of serious gravity and professional importance of a quack medical doctor giving *particular* directions for the dosing of the placebo he is leaving, he might manage to make a sound vertebra "pop." This, with his big show of doing something, has its effect on the patient's mind anyway.

We were taught that Osteopathy was applied common sense, that it was all reasonable and rational, and simply meant "finding something wrong and putting it right." Some of us thought it only fair to tell our patients what we were trying to do, and what we did it for. There is where we made our big mistake. To say we were relaxing muscles, or trying to lift and tone up a rickety chest wall, or straighten a warped spine, was altogether too simple. It was like telling a man that you were going to give him a dose of oil for the bellyache when he wanted an operation for appendicitis. It was too common, and some would go to an Osteopath who could find vertebra and ribs and hips displaced, something that would make the community "sit up and take notice." If one has to be sick, why not have something worth while?

Where Osteopathy has always been so administered that people have the idea that it means to find things out of place and put them back, it is a gentleman's job, professional, scientific and genteel. Men have been known to give twenty to forty treatments a day at two dollars per treatment. In many communities, however, the adjustment idea has so degenerated that to give an Osteopathic treatment is no job for a high collar on a hot day. To strip a hard-muscled, two-hundred-pound laborer down to a perspiration-soaked and scented undershirt, and manipulate him for an hour while he has every one of his five hundred work-hardened muscles rigidly set to protect himself from the terrible neck-wrenching, bone-twisting ordeal he has been told an Osteopathic treatment would subject him to—I say when you have tried that sort of a thing for an hour you will conclude that an Osteopathic treatment is no job for a kid-gloved dandy nor for a lily-fingered lady, as it has been so glowingly pictured.

I know the brethren will say that true Osteopathy does not give an hour's shotgun treatment, but finds the lesion, corrects it, collects its two dollars, and quits until "day after to-morrow," when it "corrects" and *collects* again as long as there is anything to co—llect!

I practiced for three years in a town where people made their first acquaintance with Osteopathy through the treatments of a man who afterwards held the position of demonstrator of Osteopathic "movements" and "manipulations" in one of the largest and boastedly superior schools of Osteopathy. The people certainly should have received correct ideas of Osteopathy from him. He was followed in the town by a bright young fellow from "Pap's" school, where the genuine "lesion," blown-in-the-bottle brand of Osteopathy has always been taught. This fellow was such an excellent Osteopath that he made enough money in two years to enable him to quit Osteopathy forever. This he did, using the money he had gathered as an Osteopath to take him through a medical college.

I followed these two shining lights who I supposed had established Osteopathy on a correct basis. I started in to give specific treatments as I had been taught to do; that is, to hunt for the lesion, correct it if I found it, and quit, even if I had not been more than fifteen or twenty minutes at it. I found that in many cases my patients were not satisfied. I did not know just what was the matter at first, and lost some desirable patients (lost their patronage, I mean—they were not in much danger of dying when they came to me). I was soon enlightened, however, by some more outspoken than the rest. They said I did not "treat as long as that other doctor," and when I had done what I thought was indicated at times a patient would say, "You didn't give me that neck-twisting movement," or that "leg-pulling treatment." No matter what I thought was indicated, I had to give all the movements each time that had ever been given before.

A physician who has had to dose out something he knew would do no good, just to satisfy the patient and keep him from sending for another doctor who he feared might give something worse, can appreciate the violence done a fellow's conscience as he administers those wonderfully curative movements. He cannot, however, appreciate the emotions that come from the strenuous exertion over a sweaty body in a close room on a July day.

Incidentally, this difference in the physical exertion necessary to get the same results has determined a good many to quit Osteopathy and take up medicine. A young man who had almost completed a course in Osteopathy told me he was going to study medicine when he had finished Osteopathy, as he had found that giving "treatments was too d———d hard work."

CHAPTER XI.

TAPEWORMS AND GALLSTONES.

Plug-hatted Faker—Frequency of Tapeworms—Some Tricks Exposed—How the Defunct Worm was Passed—Rubber Near-Worm—New Gallstone Cure—Relation to Osteopathy—Perfect, Self-Oiling, "Autotherapeutic" Machine—Touch the Button—The Truth About the Consumption and Insanity Cures.

There is another trump card the traveling medical grafter plays, which wins about as well as the guaranteed rheumatism cure, namely, the tapeworm fraud. Last summer I heard a plug-hatted faker delivering a lecture to a street crowd, in which he said that every mother's son or daughter of them who didn't have the rosy cheek, the sparkling eye and buoyancy of youth might be sure that a tapeworm of monstrous size was, "like a worm in the bud," feeding on their "damask cheeks." To prove his assertion and lend terror to his tale, he held aloft a glass jar containing one of the monsters that had been driven from its feast on the vitals of its victim by his never-failing remedy. The person, "saved from a living death," stood at the "doctor's" side to corroborate the story, while his voluptuous wife was kept busy handing out the magical remedy and "pursing the ducats" given in return.

How about the worm exhibited? How this one was secured I do not know; but intelligent people ought to know that cases of tapeworm are not so common that eight people out of every ten have one, as this grafter positively asserted.

An acquaintance once traveled with one of these tapeworm specialists to furnish the song and dance performances that are so attractive to the class of people who furnish the ready victims for grafters. This is how the game was worked. The "specialist"

92

would pick out an emaciated, credulous individual from his crowd, and tell him that he bore the unmistakable marks of being the prey of a terrible tapeworm. If he couldn't sell him a bottle of his worm eradicator, he would give him a bottle, telling him to take it according to directions and report to him at his hotel or tent the next day. The man would report that no dead or dying worm had been sighted. This was when Dr. Grafter got in his expert work. The man was told that if he had taken the medicine as directed the worm was dead beyond a doubt, but sometimes the "fangs" were fastened so firmly to the walls of the intestines, in their death agony, that they would not come away until he had injected a certain preparation that *always* "produced the goods."

The man was taken into a darkened room for privacy (?), the injection given, and the defunct worm always came away. At least a worm was always found in the evacuated material, and how was the deluded one to know that it was in the vessel or matter injected? Of course, the patient felt wondrous relief, and was glad to stand up that night and testify that Dr. Grafter was an angel of mercy sent to deliver him from the awful fate of living where "the worm dieth not and the fire is not quenched."

I was told recently of a new tapeworm graft that makes the old one look crude and unscientific. This one actually brings a tapeworm from the intestines in *every* case, whether the person had one before the magic remedy was given or not. The graft is to have a near-worm manufactured of delicate rubber and compressed into a capsule. The patient swallows the capsule supposed to contain the worm destroyer. The rubber worm is not digested, and a strong physic soon produces it, to the great relief of the "patient" and the greater glory and profit of the shyster. What a wonderful age of invention and scientific discoveries!

Another journal tells of a new gallstone cure that never fails to cause the stones to be passed even if they are big as walnuts. The graft in this is that the medicine consists of paraffine dissolved in colored oil. The paraffine does not digest, but collects in colored balls, which are passed by handfuls and are excellent imitations of the real things.

How about tapeworms, gallstones and Osteopathy, do you ask?

We heard about tapeworms and gallstones when we were in Osteopathic college.

The one thing that was ground into us early and thoroughly was that Osteopathy was a complete system. No matter what any other system had done, we were to remember that Osteopathy could do that thing more surely and more scientifically.

Students soon learned that they were never to ask, "*Can* we treat this?" That indicated skepticism, which was intolerable in the atmosphere of optimistic faith that surrounded the freshman and sophomore classes especially. The question was to be put, "*How* do we treat this?" In the treatment of worms the question was, "How do we treat worms?" That was easy. Had not nature made a machine, perfect in all its parts, self-oiling, "autotherapeutic," and all that? And would nature allow it to choke up or slip a cog just because a little thing like a worm got tangled in its gearing? Not much. Nature knew that worms would intrude, and had provided her own vermifuge. The cause of worms is insufficient bile, and behold, all the Osteopath had to do when he wished to serve notice on the aforesaid worms to vacate the premises was to touch the button controlling the stop-cock to the bile-duct, and they left. It was so simple and easy we wondered how the world could have been so long finding it out.

Osteopathy was complete. That was the proposition on which we were to stand. If anything had to be removed, or brought back, or put in place, all that was necessary was to open the floodgates, release the pent-up forces of nature, and the thing was done!

What a happy condition, to have *perfect* faith! I remember a report came to our school of an Osteopathic physician who read a paper before a convention of his brethren, in which he recorded marvelous cures performed in cases of tuberculosis. The paper was startling, even revolutionary, yet it was not too much for our faith. We were almost indignant at some who ventured to suggest that curing consumption by manipulation might be claiming too much. These wonderful cures were performed in a town which I afterward visited. I could find no one who knew of a single case that had been cured. There were those who knew of cases of tuberculosis he had treated, that had gone as most other bad cases of that disease go.

There was another world-startling case. It is one of the main cases, from all that I can learn, upon which all the bold claims of Osteopathy as an insanity cure are based. I remember an article under scare headlines big enough for a bloody murder, flared out in the local paper. It was yet more wonderfully heralded in the papers at the county seat. The metropolitan dailies caught up the echo, which reverberated through Canada and was finally heard across the seas! Osteopathic journals took it up and made much of it. Those in school read it with eager satisfaction, and plunged into their studies with fiercer enthusiasm. Many who had been "almost persuaded" were induced by it to "cross the Rubicon," and take up the study of this wonderful new science that could take a raving maniac, condemned to a mad house by medical men, and with a few scientific twists of the neck cause raging insanity to give place to gentle sleep that should wake in sanity and health.

Was it any wonder that students flocked to schools that professed to teach how common plodding mortals could work such miracles? Was it strange that anxious friends brought dear ones, over whom the black cloud of insanity cast its shadows, hundreds of miles to be treated by this man? Or to the Osteopathic colleges, from which, in all cases of which I ever knew, they returned sadly disappointed?

The report of that wonderful cure caused many intelligent laymen (and even Dr. Pratt) to indulge a hope that insanity might be only a disturbance of the blood supply to the brain caused by pressure from distorted "neck bones," or other lesions, and that Osteopaths were to empty our overcrowded madhouses. Where is that hope now? What was its foundation? I was told by an intimate friend of this great Osteopath that all these startling reports we had supposed were published as news the papers were glad to get because of their important truths, were but shrewd advertising. I afterward talked with the man, and his friends who were at the bedside when the miracle was performed, and while they believed that there had been good done by the treatment, it was all so tame and commonplace at home compared with its fame abroad that I have wondered ever since if anything much was really done after all.

THE MORAL TO THE TALE.

Honesty—Plain Dealing—Education.

But I must close. I could multiply incidents, but it would grow monotonous. I believe I have told enough that is disgusting to the intelligent laity and medical men, and enough that is humiliating to the capable, honest Osteopath, who practices his "new science" as standing for all that is good in physio-therapy.

I hope I have told, or recalled, something that will help physicians to see that the way to clear up the turbidity existing in therapeutics to-day is by open, honest dealing with the laity, and by a campaign of education that shall impart to them enough of the scientific principles of medicine so that they may know when they are being imposed upon by quacks and grafters. I am encouraged to believe I am on the right track. After I had written this booklet I read, in a report of the convention of the American Medical Association held in Chicago, that one of the leaders of the Association told his brethren that the most important work before them as physicians was to conduct a campaign of education for the masses. It must be done not only to protect the people, but as well to protect the honest physician.

There is another fact that faces the medical profession, and I believe I have called attention to conditions that prove it. That is, that the hope of the profession of "doctoring" being placed on an honest rational basis lies in a broader and more thorough education of the physician. A broad, liberal general education to begin with, then all that can be known about medicine and surgery. Is that enough? No. Then all that there is in physio-therapy, under whatsoever name, that promises to aid in curing or preventing disease.

If this humble production aids but a little in any of this great work, then my object in writing will have been achieved.

www.ingramcontent.com/pod-product-compliance
Lightning Source LLC
Chambersburg PA
CBHW051342170526
45166CB00002B/915